Type 2 Diabetes in Teens

Secrets for Success

**Jean Betschart-Roemer,
MN, MSN, CPNP, CDE**

John Wiley & Sons, Inc.

Published by John Wiley & Sons, Inc., New York
Published simultaneously in Canada

This publication is designed to provide accurate and authoritative information in regard to the subject matter covered. It is sold with the understanding that the publisher is not engaged in rendering professional services. If professional advice or other expert assistance is required, the services of a competent professional person should be sought.

Wiley also publishes its books in a variety of electronic formats. Some content that appears in print may not be available in electronic books. For more information about Wiley products, visit our web site at www.wiley.com.

ISBN 0-471-15056-8

Printed in the United States of America

10 9 8 7 6 5 4 3 2 1

Contents

Acknowledgments

I wish to thank my friends and colleagues at the Children's Hospital of Pittsburgh Diabetes Center who supported and encouraged the writing of this book. I also give special thanks to the teens who took time to participate by sharing their thoughts, feelings, and helpful ideas so that others can benefit.

Family and friends are precious to me, and the writing of this work has cost me time away from them. I thank Bill, and my family and friends, for encouragement and understanding of time spent on this project. And finally, I thank God for His constant blessings and the privileges given to me, such as this opportunity to write.

Love,

Jean

Introduction

Five or ten years ago, there would have been a very limited market for this book. Things have changed in a very short period of time!

Part of the reason for this change is due to the tremendous effort in diabetes research promoted by both the American Diabetes Association and the Juvenile Diabetes Research Foundation, International. Substantial amounts of money are being donated to diabetes research efforts, which are both clarifying and complicating the diagnosis of diabetes. As it turns out, some children and teens who have been diagnosed with type 1 diabetes over the years may in fact have type *2* diabetes! Of course, the treatment for both is to keep blood glucose levels as close to normal as possible, but the understanding and strategy for doing that might be somewhat different. The increase of type 2 diabetes in children and teens is partially due to the fact that it is being recognized and diagnosed more readily, and also to the increasing incidence of type 2 diabetes in the general population.

Families and health professionals alike often confuse the course and treatment of type 1 and type 2 diabetes, leaving a teen not knowing where to begin to ask questions. Sometimes teens, parents, and others are told that they have "a touch" of diabetes or "borderline" diabetes. What this usually means is that there are few, if any, obvious symptoms of high blood sugar but that blood sugar may at times run higher than normal. They do not have overt clinical diabetes, but may have abnormal blood glucose or insulin levels produced in response to food. The test that measures this is called a *glucose tolerance test*. When tested, a person is given an exact amount of something sweet to drink and blood sugar and insulin levels are then measured at specific times and compared to normal. It is possible to have abnormal glucose regulation, yet not have any clinical or sub-clinical signs of diabetes.

Teens with type 2 diabetes may not fully understand the seriousness of diabetes, the importance of treatment, and/or how to care for themselves. Often a teen is told to lose weight but given little help on exactly how to do it. Family members may not have a clear understanding of the issues or may have misinformation about what is required. In particular, teens who have type 2 diabetes may not take their disease seriously. This concerns me a great deal as this contributes to poor diabetes control, and, ultimately, unnecessary complications of diabetes.

As a nurse practitioner and diabetes educator who works daily with children and teens with diabetes, I personally know that there is a need for educational materials designed just to help a teen with type 2 diabetes. Of the flyers, booklets, books, and leaflets on diabetes available for people with type 2 diabetes, none of them, as of this writing, specifically address the special needs and situations of a teenager. Most of what is written for children and teens with diabetes is intended for those with type 1 diabetes, and although some of the information can be applied to both kinds of diabetes, there are distinct differences between the two types. Other materials written for people with type 2 diabetes are focused on adult issues.

As an educator and health care professional who has specialized in development and health promotion, my job is to teach children, teens, their families, and their friends what they need to know to take good care of themselves. As there are few resources to allow a teen with type 2 to reinforce her learning and keep her motivated, I wanted to provide a book that is positive, sympathetic, informative, and motivational. I wanted to offer a book that explains diabetes care in terms that a teen can understand and that talks about issues such as drinking, driving, substance abuse, sexuality, pregnancy, college, sports, dating, depression, complications, and other issues as they relate to type 2 diabetes.

I know a lot about the subject from both personal and professional experiences. I was diagnosed with type 1 at the age of 19. Additionally, I grew up as an overweight child and teen, and have been battling to control my weight all my life. I know what it feels like to be overweight and sedentary. I know what it feels like to have high and low blood glucose levels, monitor blood glucose, and do all of the things that someone with type 2 diabetes must do. Although I cannot relate to growing up with type 2 diabetes, I have personal experience with many of the issues. Most of what I have learned about dealing with type 2 diabetes, however, comes from talks with teens, who never fail to teach me.

As a teen with diabetes, you should have an understanding of what is going on in your body and what can be done about it. You need to feel as though you can do what you need to do to live a long and healthy life. Knowledge is key to your treatment. Then comes the hard part of translating what you know into the health practices that you do every day. I hope that this book does all of that, and helps to motivate you to love and take care of yourself. Take care, and good luck!

I put the finishing touches on this book September 11, 2001. As a nurse practitioner, I have dedicated my life to fostering wellness and health promotion, and find it ironic to complete this book on the very day of the national disaster this country has seen today. With angst in my heart, I dedicate this book to all who have lost their lives, and those who are in pain, who are grieving, and who have been affected by senseless terrorism.

1

What's Happening to Me?

Maria's Story

Maria sat on the exam table while her mother relaxed in the nearby chair. She felt really tired and a bit thirsty. She hadn't slept well because she had been up going to the bathroom all night long. Then thirst would send her searching for big glasses of ice water and soda. She had been so tired she barely could make the effort to comb her thick dark hair, and then she almost missed her bus! Now she felt scrubby and irritable. She was tired of waiting, had already finished her homework, and wanted to go hang out with some friends. After all, they had been in the doctor's office a long time and it was a beautiful day outside. She took another sip of her drink and wondered why she was so thirsty in spite of having just drunk two cans of soda.

It was now almost spring, but she remembered that she had started being thirsty off and on since last summer, the summer of her fourteenth birthday. Uncle Carlos and Aunt Juanita had a surprise party for her, and she smiled when she remembered how much cake and other treats she had eaten that day. ("If anyone found out, I'd be so embarrassed!") Afterward was the first time she noticed the extreme thirst and dry mouth. At first she thought the thirst was just because she was sweating in the summer heat, but the thirst never completely went away. She noticed that the thirst seemed worse after she ate a big meal. Then, lately, she was getting up to go to the bathroom a couple of times a night. A few weeks ago when she came home from school, after having had a baking fair in cooking class, she went to the sink and drank five glasses of water. Mama stood by watching, then spoke in Spanish, saying, "Maria, I think something is wrong. You just shouldn't be drinking that much. I'm going to make a doctor's appointment for you."

So here they were, waiting and waiting. Maria wondered if something was wrong because although she had been eating quite a lot lately, she hadn't gained any weight. Actually the nurse had told her that her weight was down a few pounds. She thought that was pretty great, because as long as she could remember, she'd been trying to lose weight. Diets had never worked before. Although she could lose a few pounds from time to time, she never could keep it off, and pretty soon she'd gain it all back. But now she was eating more than ever, and had actually lost weight! Lately she had noticed she was more likely to drink a lot than be hungry for food.

Eat this, don't eat that! It felt like everyone was always on her case. At her physical exam in school last fall, she remembered how her school nurse had frowned, saying, "Maria, your weight is up even more than last year." "Well, look at my family!" she responded. In her whole family, no one was thin. How could they expect her to weigh less than her overweight family? "Besides," she thought, "I don't really eat that much most of the time."

Dr. Lanai now came into the room looking very serious. He was a tall man with short gray hair, and he usually kidded around with her. But today, there were no jokes. "Maria, I just tested the urine sample you gave us and found out that you have a lot of sugar in your urine. I think that you have diabetes, so we're going to have to do some *more tests. I'm going to send you over to the hospital for some blood work."*

Maria had no idea what he was talking about. She groaned and thought that she'd really be late now for getting together with her friends. Although her grandmother, her uncle, and a cousin had diabetes, she had never paid much attention to it. Actually, she felt a little bit scared now, and even Mama looked worried. Dr. Lanai said, "I'm sorry, Maria. Let's wait to see what your blood tests show . . ."

Diabetes Is on the Rise!

The number of people who have diabetes in the United States and in the world is increasing. There is a lot of research being done on why this is so, but one of the main reasons is that people are more overweight than ever before, and that includes children and teens. People today are less active, spend more time in front of the television and computer, eat more fast foods, eat larger portions, and drink more sugary beverages than at any other time in history! All of these habits have caused people to gain too much weight. And being overweight and inactive contributes to the number of teens who develop type 2 diabetes.

Type 2 diabetes occurs more often in people with certain ethnic backgrounds. People who are of African-American, Hispanic, and American Indian backgrounds are at additional risk. Although young children can develop type 2 diabetes, it is most commonly diagnosed in children around the age of 13 or 14. Recent studies have found that type 2 diabetes makes up about 16 to 30 percent of the new cases of diabetes in children between the ages of 10 and 19. Experts are in agreement that this number is rising all the time.

Bottom Line

More children and teens are being diagnosed with type 2 diabetes than ever before.

Maria's Story

Maria and her mom were waiting again, this time in the admissions office of the hospital. Dr. Lanai had called with the results of her tests and said that she should come into the hospital for a few days. He explained that they needed her to go into the hospital to get her blood sugar under control, decide how to best treat the diabetes, and teach her how to take care of herself.

So Maria had packed a few things, picked up her homework, and gone back to the hospital. She now wondered why she had to be there. She and Mama walked into her hospital room, where nurses greeted her and introduced Sally, a "diabetes nurse educator." Maria had never heard of a diabetes educator before. Sally explained that she was a nurse whose job it was to teach them about diabetes and how to manage it. Maria looked at Mama, who now was looking like she was going to cry. Maybe this whole thing was more serious than she thought. Maybe she should forget about her afterschool activities and homework. Maybe she was going to die! All of a sudden Maria had a terrible feeling in her stomach.

Sally was very kind and patient as she talked to Maria and her mother, but Maria was basically zoning out; after all, she had been thinking about dying! Suddenly she heard Sally ask, "Do you have any questions for now?"

Maria's friends and family sometimes teased her about being too direct, to the point of being blunt. Maria usually said what was on her mind. So, characteristically, Maria blurted out her thought: "Am I going to die?"

Sally smiled gently and gave her hand a pat. "No, Maria!

Of course everyone is going to die sooner or later, but you can control diabetes and live a long, healthy life. In fact, you can do anything you want to do with your life if you take care of yourself. But you will have to do some things that other kids don't have to do. You will need to lose weight, exercise, and live a healthy lifestyle. Sometimes the things that you must do are hard, but I am here to teach you what to do. Your family will help you, too. We'll be talking about what happens when you get diabetes, and how you can take care of yourself." Maria suddenly felt like doing two things: calling her best friend, Rita, and praying.

The next morning, Maria, her parents, her brother, Roberto, and Rita all met around a table in Sally's office. It was the beginning of this process of diabetes education that everyone talked about. Maria groaned inwardly and felt like she didn't want to do any of it. She was tired and wanted to go back to bed, but since everyone was here, she figured she might as well do what she had to so she could get out of there. "It sounds like a hassle," she thought, "but at least I'm not going to die." Sally began teaching.

Inside Workings

Some people think that science is boring. But when you have diabetes, it is important to understand what is going on in your body so that you can make good decisions about your care. So try to focus for a minute to learn how your body normally works (see Figure 1).

The pancreas is an organ that is tucked near your stomach. It makes digestive juice, and other hormones. About 10 percent of the cells in the pancreas make a hormone called *insulin*. When you eat or drink something, the stomach turns the food or liquid into glucose, a form of sugar. The glucose goes into your bloodstream and travels throughout your body, feeding body cells so they can have energy. With enough energy, a cell can do everything it *should* do!

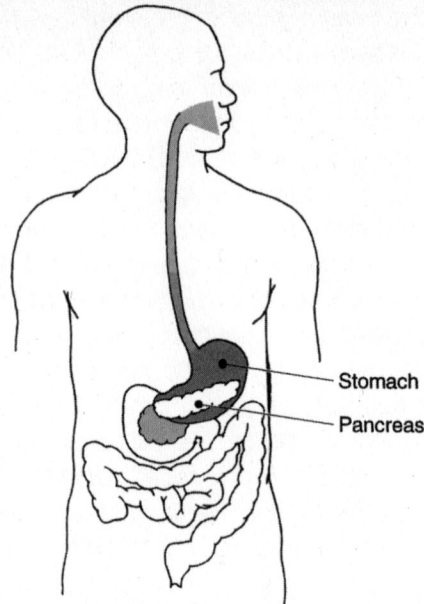

Figure 1: Where your pancreas is located.

For example, a brain cell helps you think and governs your whole body. A blood cell travels and may carry nutrients to other cells or fight off infections. A muscle cell gives you strength. Cells in your lungs help you breathe. The hormone insulin that the pancreas produces works like a key does in unlocking a lock: it unlocks the "doors" to the cells, allowing the glucose to go inside and do its work (see Figure 2). Without glucose, the cells do not work well. If there is enough glucose and insulin in your body, the cells are fed. However, if there isn't enough glucose or insulin, or if the insulin has a problem unlocking the door to the cells, the cells cannot get food, and your body will not have the energy it needs to get things done (see Figure 3).

Bottom Line

Insulin delivers sugar (glucose) to body cells.

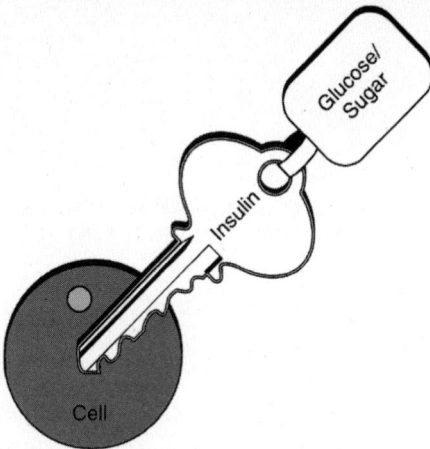

Figure 2: Cell getting sugar through insulin.

Maria's Story

Sally drew explanatory pictures while she talked. Although Maria was a little tired of sitting, she actually found this lesson interesting. Mr. Standish, her biology teacher, had shown her cells under a microscope. She had done well on the test on which she had to identify the parts of a cell. She remembered the words "cell wall," "receptor," and even "mitochondria." She remembered something about needing fuel to burn for energy. She was impressed that she remembered this stuff!

Maria wondered, "What does this all have to do with me?" As if reading her mind, Sally said, "Now, you're probably wondering what this means for you . . ."

How Diabetes Affects Your Body

When the glucose cannot get into the cells of the body to give them energy, it begins to build up in the bloodstream. Then there is a high level of sugar in the blood. Some of the sugar is filtered out through the kidneys and into the urine. Therefore, people with high blood sugar also have sugar in their urine.

The sugar molecule is heavy, though, so when it is pulled out

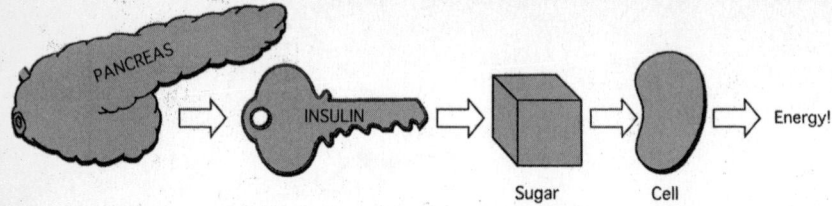

Figure 3: Normally the pancreas makes insulin that unlocks the door to cells that allows them to use sugar for energy.

into the urine, it takes a large volume of water with it. This makes for a large amount of urine, so you have to go to the bathroom a lot. Sometimes the need to urinate a lot is most noticeable during the night. You may then become more dehydrated, and begin to drink because you're thirsty. And, of course, when you drink a lot, it makes for large volumes of urine. When you lose a lot of water in the urine, it pulls other things your body needs with it, such as sodium and potassium. And being dehydrated makes you feel tired (see Figure 4).

Also, having high blood sugar in your body makes things that you look at appear blurry. High blood sugar also causes your wounds not to heal quickly, and sometimes they can become infected. Sometimes you lose weight because the food you eat is not being used properly by your body. Instead, the calories are lost in your urine. All of the following are signs of diabetes:

- Increased urination
- Increased thirst
- Increased hunger
- Weight loss
- Blurred vision
- Infections
- Wounds or cuts that don't heal

Bottom Line

The signs of diabetes occur because there is *too much sugar* in the blood, or high blood sugar.

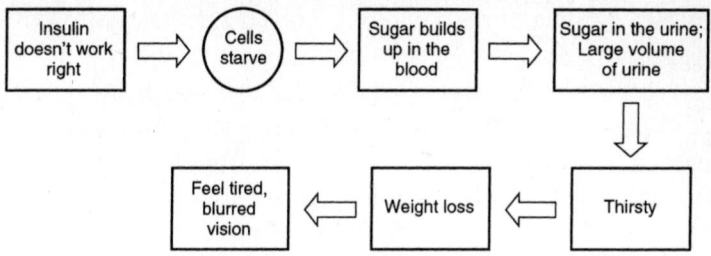

Figure 4: Progression of symptoms.

Maria's Story

As Maria heard Sally's explanation, it all started to make sense. She said, "That's why I was so tired! And sometimes I was afraid I might not make it to the bathroom in time. Remember? Mama, I had that infected finger around Thanksgiving and it just wouldn't go away. And you know what else? I cut my ankle two months ago on the bottom of our screen door and it still hasn't gone away." As Sally bent over to examine Maria's ankle, Dad gave her a hug and said, "Well, we've been worried about you, Maria. You've seemed tired to us. And I never saw anyone drink so much soda." Sally straightened up, then continued, "All of this means that you have diabetes."

What are the Types of Diabetes?

Diabetes mellitus is the term that was used to describe the problem of having high blood sugar for many years. Until the twentieth century there was no understanding that there were different types of diabetes, or even exactly what caused high blood sugar. Diabetes mellitus was recognized as a medical problem as long ago as around 30 C.E. The word "diabetes" means "to run through"; "mellitus" means "honeyed." One of the ways physicians or healers diagnosed their patients back then was to taste the urine, and if it was sweet, they knew that their patient had diabetes. Thankfully, we have more sophisticated tools to test for diabetes today! Even now, however, diabetes is sometimes diagnosed as the result of a screening test on your urine. Normal urine should not have sugar in it.

For many years it was not known that there are different types of diabetes. It was thought that diabetes is diabetes! Now, however, it is known that there are different types of diabetes. Our understanding of both type 1 and type 2 diabetes is still growing, though, and it is thought that perhaps some children or teens who have been diagnosed as having type 1 may actually have type 2 diabetes. The symptoms and features of both kinds have become clearer as research has progressed. Although some people learn that it is not completely clear which type they have, for both types of diabetes the goal is *to keep blood sugar levels well controlled.* This means trying to keep blood sugar levels as close to normal (70–120 mg/dl) as possible.

Associations such as the American Diabetes Association and the Juvenile Diabetes Foundation, International are working to get the word out to health care providers and the public about what diabetes is, the different types, who is most likely to get it, the signs and symptoms, and the different treatments. Even so, there is a lot more work to do because most people do not understand the differences between the different types of diabetes. So sometimes you may have to be responsible for explaining it to others yourself! Here are some important facts about type 1 and type 2 diabetes. We'll cover this information in more detail in the sections that follow.

Type 1 Diabetes

➤ Can occur at any age, but is the most common form in children, teens, and young adults.

➤ Is an *autoimmune* (explained below) disease.

➤ Ketones in the urine are common. Ketones are a waste product made when the body burns fat for energy. This happens when cells are starving due to there not being enough insulin.

➤ Requires insulin for treatment.

➤ Teens and children are usually normal weight.

Type 2 Diabetes

➢ Can occur at any age, but is the most common form of diabetes in adults.

➢ There is insulin resistance. This means the insulin that is present doesn't work well.

➢ Treatment may be diet, exercise, pills, and/or insulin.

➢ Teens and others are usually overweight.

➢ It runs more in families than type #1.

TYPE 1 DIABETES

Type 1 diabetes is what is known as an *autoimmune disease*. *Auto* means "self." Your immune system is made of fighting cells, which protect you from a cold, flu, or other illness. However, in an autoimmune disease, your own immune system attacks and destroys a part of your own body.

In type 1 diabetes, fighting cells, called *antibodies,* attack the islet cells in the pancreas, which make insulin. This means that in this kind of diabetes, no more insulin can be made because the cells that make the insulin are destroyed. So a person must take insulin in some other way: by syringe, pen, pump, or possibly an inhaler. Type 1 diabetes used to be called *juvenile diabetes* or *insulin-dependent diabetes mellitus* (IDDM); these terms are not used anymore.

Most children and teens who develop diabetes get type 1 diabetes. It usually comes on suddenly, with symptoms increasing over a period of a few days, weeks, or months. Children can get very sick very quickly, and may start vomiting. Sometimes this kind of diabetes is mistaken for the flu when it first comes on because some of the symptoms are flu-like. Diabetes often can follow the flu or a viral infection.

Scientists have now pinpointed the genes for type 1 diabetes, and are able to predict pretty accurately who might get it from their gene types. You inherit genes from all of your ancestors. Therefore, type 1 diabetes can run in families.

Bottom Line

Type 1 diabetes is a disease in which the pancreas makes little or no insulin because the cells that make insulin have been destroyed.

TYPE 2 DIABETES

Type 2 diabetes is the most common type of diabetes in adults and is now starting to show up more and more in younger people like you! It used to be called *maturity-onset diabetes, adult-onset diabetes,* and *non-insulin-dependent diabetes* (NIDDM); these terms are no longer used. A person with this type of diabetes might have plenty of insulin being made, but the body cannot use it properly. The insulin being made doesn't work, and over time, the constant stress of overproducing insulin so that the cells can get food causes the cells that make insulin to burn out. Then there is little insulin being made, and what is there doesn't work. Like a person with type 1, the person with type 2 diabetes might need to take insulin in a syringe or by some other means, but this still does not mean that they have type 1 diabetes.

Type 2 diabetes is often unrecognized. This happens because type 2 diabetes can come on slowly. The American Diabetes Association estimates that there are millions of people in the United States who have undiagnosed diabetes. People can have type 2 diabetes for a very long time and not know it, because the symptoms come on so gradually. Sometimes there are no symptoms at all, and the first thing to show up is a complication of diabetes! (See Chapter 4, "Preventing Complications.")

What is a complication? Well, when you begin to develop type 2 diabetes, sometimes the level of sugar in your blood might be too high but you may not have any signs of high blood sugar. You may not notice any problem and not know that you have diabetes until complications begin. A complication is a problem with the eyes, nerves, kidneys, or blood vessels, caused by high blood sugar levels over a long period of time. For this reason it is good to diagnose diabetes and treat it early in order to prevent or delay complications. If there is any suspicion that diabetes is present, it is very smart to be checked.

Let's talk a little more about the workings of type 2 diabetes. As you know, glucose is a form of sugar. Cells in the body use insulin to get glucose for energy. In type 2 diabetes, the insulin doesn't work properly to get glucose into the cells. If you think of insulin as being a key that unlocks the door in the cell wall to let insulin inside, what happens in type 2 diabetes is that the key doesn't fit the lock. This is called *insulin resistance.* The cells are *resistant* to insulin's action. This is a very important term to know.

Bottom Line

Type 2 diabetes occurs when the insulin doesn't work properly and/or there isn't enough insulin.

When you are a teen, your body makes a lot of hormones, which are chemicals released from body organs into the bloodstream. Everyone has certain hormones that are necessary for life. But teens have extra hormones that cause them to grow, and develop into a man or woman. These hormones regulate growth, development, and sexual functioning. These hormones also cause insulin resistance. In addition, being overweight and inactive makes insulin resistance worse. Plus, if anyone has type 2 diabetes in your family, you are more at risk for getting it yourself. So if that is the case, it is smart to be proactive and do what you can do to prevent it from happening.

When someone who is overweight loses weight and exercises, the insulin can do its job better, and blood sugar improves. You will need to exercise more, as today people tend to weigh more and exercise less. And there's a good explanation for why this is so.

Years ago, back in the days when life was very, very primitive, those who were strongest and had the most meat on their bones were the people who survived against starvation and the other forces of nature. When there was no food or bitter cold, the people who survived were those who had a body that was very efficient, and who could live on very little food. Over many generations, man's body adapted by developing what is now sometimes called a "thrifty gene." People who have this do not burn food easily and can survive on a small number of calories. Sometimes you will hear people call this a "slow metabolism." These folks don't need many calories to maintain their weight, since their body uses food very efficiently. This might be the case with you! In the old days, you would have been one to survive cold temperatures, drought, and famine!

Years ago, or even as recently as the era in which your grandparents and great-grandparents lived, people had to be more active in their daily life than today. Today we don't have to wash clothes by hand. We don't have to go hunting to bring home dinner. Almost everyone has a car, so people don't walk much. In fact, most people look for the parking space closest to their destination so that they don't have to walk too far! Think of all the times in a day you might use technology that your ancestors didn't have. You don't have to knead the dough to have daily bread; you don't have to run up the street to see a neighbor, but can call on the phone; you don't have to turn the knob on the can opener because the electric one is easy; you don't have to beat the rug in your room to clean it because you have a vacuum cleaner; you don't have to walk stairs because you take the elevator! Now that television exists, people spend an average of two to three hours a day watching TV rather than farming the land or doing some other activity that uses calories and burns fat. With a remote, you don't even have to get up out of your chair to shut off the TV! We are far less active today than our ancestors, who had more exercise and less food! It is no wonder that people are gaining weight, and that, as we've already seen, makes us more at risk for diabetes and other diseases.

So part of the fault of diabetes-on-the-rise belongs to our society. But also, some of the fault belongs to the individual. We

> ### Bottom Line
>
> You can cut your risk of getting type 2 diabetes by keeping a healthy body weight and exercising!

can blame our extra weight gain on today's culture, but that is an explanation, not an excuse! Everyone is responsible for their own health and well-being, and that means that you are, too!

OTHER TYPES OF DIABETES

There are other types of diabetes that are not as common as type 1 or type 2 diabetes. One type is called *gestational diabetes mellitus* (GDM), and occurs in women who are pregnant. It is extremely important for women with GDM to control their blood glucose during pregnancy so they can have a healthy baby. This kind of diabetes usually goes away after the baby is born, but women who have it are more at risk then for developing type 2 diabetes.

Diabetes can also be caused by injury or disease in the pancreas (remember that organ we talked about that makes insulin? See page 8), or a defect in the genes that make or use insulin. Some drugs and chemicals can also cause diabetes. This kind of diabetes is called *secondary diabetes,* meaning that the diabetes was due to some other problem. For example, teens who have had organ transplants and are on drugs to keep their body from rejecting the organ can get diabetes from the drugs they are on. Steroids can also cause high blood sugar. In these cases, if the teen is able to stop taking the drugs or chemicals causing high blood sugar, the blood sugar level might go back to normal and the person might no longer have diabetes.

Bottom Line

Blood glucose levels are high in all types of diabetes. However, there are varied reasons why the high blood sugar occurs.

Maria's Story

She was definitely ready to get out of there. She needed to go to the restroom and get a drink. Besides that, she was hungry. This morning's breakfast had been even larger than usual, but it seemed that no matter what she ate, she was always hungry. Sally sensed her restlessness and said, "Okay, why don't we take a twenty-minute break."

As they walked back to her room, they saw Dr. Lanai walking toward them. "I was looking for you! How are things going?"

Maria suspected that he already knew how things were going, but she decided not to be smart. "Okay. Well, I found out that my blood sugar was high all night."

"I know," he murmured. "If you have a few minutes, I'd like to talk to you." Maria and her parents went into her room, while Rita and Roberto decided to go get a drink.

"Maria, I'm not completely certain yet, but I suspect that you have type 2 diabetes. You've probably had the signs for a year. You already have type 2 diabetes in your family, and you are overweight. The word is actually obese, but I know that beautiful young women like you don't like that word." He smiled kindly at her. "Whichever type it is, however, you are going to start taking insulin. Sally will teach you how to give yourself an injection. After you take insulin and get onto a healthy plan of eating, we are hoping that you will lose weight and might eventually be able to go off taking the insulin shots. I can't make any promises, but the best thing you can do for yourself, young lady, is to lose weight. Terry, our dietitian, will meet with

you and teach you what needs to be done. It is never easy to lose weight, but I believe you can do it!"

Maria listened carefully, then said, "Well, I'd like to lose weight. I've always hated being fat, but I just never could lose weight. Maybe I don't know how."

Mama spoke up with her soft accent. "Well, we will all help. Maybe we can do it with you. We can all afford to lose some weight. Even Roberto! So I think we should do it as a family. It will be good for all of us!"

Roberto walked in the room at that moment and stopped in his tracks. "What do you mean?" he grumbled. "I don't have to go on a diet. I don't have diabetes. Why should I be deprived of food just because she can't have it?"

Hmmm . . .

What Happens Next?

It's important to learn as much as you can about your diabetes, and that includes an understanding of what kind of diabetes you have. It may not be obvious to your doctors at first, but with some extra tests, it can become clearer. The most important thing to remember is that no matter what kind of diabetes you have, the treatment is to keep blood sugar levels *as normal as possible*. And that is done by doing whatever it takes to keep them normal. You will learn to control your diabetes, and develop healthy eating and exercise habits so that you can live a healthy life.

2

How to Control Diabetes— and Feel Great! Seven Steps

Maria's Story

After lunch, they all met in Sally's office again. This time, Sally had bottles of insulin, bottles of saline (salt water), and syringes on the table. Maria wondered how she'd ever be able to give herself a shot. She remembered when she had had shots in the past, such as vaccinations and penicillin, and how they had hurt. Again, as if reading her mind, Sally softly said, "Shots that you've had before might have hurt a lot, but I think you'll find that these needles are so fine they don't hurt much, and the insulin doesn't burn going in. But before we get into giving injections, we need to go over a few more things."

Treating Type 2 Diabetes

If you or your parents bought this book, chances are you have Type 2 diabetes. So let's concentrate on this type. It is most important that you understand what diabetes is and know the things you can do to take care of it. The following are steps you can take that will lead you to good health. The rest of this chapter will explain what you need to know for all of the steps.

Seven Steps to Treat Your Type 2 Diabetes

1. Understand what type 2 diabetes is.
2. Find a doctor or health care team who is experienced in treating teens with diabetes.
3. Learn to test your blood sugar, and do it often!
4. Take medication regularly, and on time, if you need it.
5. Watch for signs of low blood sugar.
6. Eat healthy and maintain a healthy weight.
7. Exercise!

Step #1: Understand What Type 2 Diabetes Is

People with type 2 diabetes can have a double problem: Not only doesn't insulin work well, but there may not be enough of it, at least not enough for an overweight body. (How much insulin you need is directly related to how much you weigh.) These two problems also cause the liver to release too much glucose, so your blood sugar is high. As you lose weight, however, which you do through diet and exercise, and as your blood glucose level improves, the insulin can begin to work better in your body. In other words, your body becomes more sensitive to the action of the insulin.

Your goal is to keep your blood sugar under the best possible control. The ways of doing this are by healthy eating, exercise, weight loss, and, yes, medication. If your blood sugar can be well controlled with healthy eating, exercise, and weight loss, you might not even need medication. But if those aren't doing the trick, then you may need to add a pill. And if your blood sugar still runs very high, you may need to take insulin.

It is important to remember that just because you need insulin at first, it does not necessarily mean that you will always need insulin. Sometimes when diabetes is newly diagnosed, you may need insulin. Then, as your blood sugar control improves through watching your diet, exercising, and losing weight, your insulin works better and you may need less of it. And sometimes a teen might not need any insulin and have very normal blood sugar! That doesn't mean, however, that the diabetes is cured. It can come back during times of stress, when you fall off your healthy eating plan, or if you gain weight.

Try to get into your head a mind-set that you need to do "whatever it takes!" As you've just read, the goal is to keep the blood sugar level as normal as possible. So if it takes diet and exercise, that's great! But if it takes pills and insulin, too, well, yes, that's a little more complicated, but you've got to do it to be able to reach your goal. When you have diabetes, keeping a normal blood sugar level is the most important thing you can do for your health.

Bottom Line

The best treatment for type 2 diabetes is a combination of a healthy diet, exercise, pills, and/or insulin.

Step #2: Find a Doctor or Health Care Team Who Is Experienced in Treating Teens with Diabetes

When you have diabetes and are a teen, it is important that your health care professionals are expert in dealing with teens with diabetes. Although diabetes care teams are excellent places to go when you have diabetes, many people do not live in places where a team is readily available. Because children and teens with diabetes have their own unique problems, they usually do best when their treatment is followed by a diabetes care team of professionals. These multidisciplinary teams are most often found in major medical centers. There are also pediatric centers equipped to follow teens through their graduation from high school, and many will continue beyond that.

Since type 2 diabetes used to be called "maturity" or "adult-onset" diabetes, some people still feel that since teens with type 2 have the "adult" form of the disease, a doctor who sees adults should follow them. However, teens have their own issues, separate from adults, and should go somewhere where the medical care team is experienced and suitable for the special needs of teens. Adolescent medicine is its own specialty, and teens with diabetes are no exception.

One of the first things to do is to ask your health care provider for the names of doctors or centers recommended in your location. Think about whether the recommended doctor is a specialist in diabetes. If you are lucky enough to live near a major diabetes center, there may be a team of diabetes specialists and other team members available to you. Sometimes the doctor who diagnoses your diabetes will be the one you continue to go to, and other times the doctor may refer you to a diabetes care team of professionals. You may find a doctor in private practice and, with help, might put together your own team of health professionals, including a diabetes educator and a dietitian.

WHO'S ON YOUR TEAM?

It is important to understand who the people on your team are and what they do. If you don't know, you can ask them!

Types of health care professionals who might be on your team:

Diabetologist—a doctor (M.D., D.O.) who specializes in treating patients with diabetes

Endocrinologist—a doctor (M.D, D.O.) who specializes in treating hormone imbalances, which includes diabetes

Family Practitioner—a primary care doctor (M.D., D.O.) who treats a wide variety of conditions in children and adults

General Practitioner—a primary care doctor (M.D., D.O.) who treats a wide variety of conditions in adults

Internist—a doctor (M.D., D.O.) who has specialized in medical diseases, including diabetes

Pediatrician—a primary care doctor (M.D., D.O.) who treats children and teens

Pediatric Endocrinologist—a pediatrician (M.D., D.O.) who has extra training in the study of hormones

Ophthalmologist—a medical doctor (M.D., D.O.) who has specialty training in diseases of the eyes. Eye problems can be a complication of diabetes.

Nephrologist—a medical doctor (M.D., D.O.) who has specialty training in diseases of the kidney. Kidney disease can be a complication of diabetes.

Neurologist—a medical doctor (M.D., D.O.) who has specialty training in diseases of the nerves. Nerve disease can be a complication of diabetes.

Podiatrist—a doctor (D.P.M.) who is trained to take care of conditions of the feet, which can suffer complications caused by diabetes

Psychiatrist/Psychologist—a doctor (M.D. or Ph.D.) who is an expert in behavioral science and who can counsel you if you are having trouble dealing with any part of your diabetes

Dentist—a doctor (D.M.D.) who is trained to take care of diseases and conditions of the teeth, mouth, and gums

Certified Diabetes Educator (C.D.E.)—a registered nurse, dietitian, social worker, pharmacist, exercise physiologist, doctor, or other licensed health professional who has passed a national exam on diabetes education and care

Nurse Educator—a nurse who will teach you how to monitor your blood sugar, take medication, treat low blood sugar, and manage your blood sugar for special activities

Social Worker (L.S.W.)—a licensed health professional who can give you information about diabetes services, medical care, resources, and support. A social worker can guide you to where you might find financial help, or provide counseling services.

Registered Dietitian (R.D.)—a licensed health professional who can help with a healthy eating plan, and will guide and encourage you in your weight loss efforts

Exercise Physiologist—a licensed health professional who can guide you into an exercise program and give you encouragement to help you lose weight and become physically fit

WHO ELSE IS ON THE TEAM?

You and your parents!

In fact, not only are you on the team, you are the *center* of it! The people who gather to be on your team are your guides and your cheerleaders. They are the people whose job it is to help YOU take care of yourself. They have knowledge, training, and experience in their specialty. You have knowledge, training, and experience in YOU! So everyone must share their information to have the best outcome.

Diabetes is obviously not a disease where your doctor can give you a treatment, you are cured, and you can go home and forget about it. Your treatment is actually up to *you.* So it is very important that you surround yourself with people who are able and willing to help.

Maria's Story

Maria was putting together a list of her own team already when Sally suggested that she think about it. There'd be Mama, Papa, Grandmama, Rita, and, well, okay, maybe Roberto. Then there would be Uncle Carlos, Juanita, Mr. Santiago, her biology teacher and one of her favorites, and Mrs. Julio, the drill team coach. Dr. Lanai would be a definite . . .

Step #3: Learn to Test Your Blood Sugar, and Do It Often!

Because keeping blood sugar as close to normal as possible is the goal of your treatment, it is important to know how high or low your blood sugar is. People with diabetes must test, or monitor, their blood glucose regularly so that they can make smart decisions in their diabetes care. Teens with type 2 diabetes are no exception, and many excellent products today can help you do just that. In fact, blood glucose monitoring is easier than ever before, with new products being developed all the time!

As a teen, you will most likely want a testing device, called a *meter,* that is easy to use, fast, inconspicuous, accurate, and has a memory. Meters with glucose level, date, and time memories are great because they retain all of your testing information. So if you forget to write it down, the date, time, and test result are still there. This record of blood sugar numbers with the date and time is really helpful when it comes time to make decisions about your treatment. A diabetes educator can show you the different meters that are available. Sometimes, however, insurance companies will only pay for certain products, so you and your parents will have to decide which meter is best for you, depending on your particular situation.

First, you'll need to meet with your doctor, who will tell you *how often* and *when* to monitor your blood sugar. The number of times a day you monitor your blood glucose will depend upon whether you are taking a pill for diabetes treatment or using insulin. People who take insulin monitor their blood glucose four times a day. Others might need to check their blood in the morning and/or after meals. It's smart to keep records of blood glucose numbers because you and your health care team can find patterns in the numbers, which may guide your treatment!

Bottom Line

Testing your blood sugar gives you information that helps you manage your diabetes.

Step #4: Take Medication Regularly, and On Time, if You Need to

You may not need pills to treat your diabetes. But if you do need medication, there are excellent new products that help to lower blood sugar. Don't be confused by thinking that they are "insulin pills." Insulin, in its current form, cannot be swallowed in pill form, because it is a protein and will be digested by the stomach just like a piece of meat! However, some pills that your doctor might prescribe for you will work by causing insulin to be made.

And some of them cause the insulin to work better. Other pills can prevent the starch in food you eat from being absorbed well. Pills that end up lowering your blood sugar are called *oral agents.* They are designed to lower blood glucose in a variety of ways. Your doctor will know which one might be the best for you. They might:

- cause your liver to cut back on the amount of sugar being released, and at the same time help the liver and muscles be more sensitive to insulin
- help the insulin to be used more efficiently
- stimulate the pancreas to make insulin
- slow down or prevent the absorption of carbohydrate in your food (more about carbohydrate later!)
- improve the action of insulin in your body cells

If your doctor gives you a pill to treat your diabetes, one of the most likely ones that children and teens use is called *metformin* (Glucophage). It is usually tried first because it does as good a job of lowering blood glucose as some of the other drugs, and yet it doesn't have the effect of causing *low* blood sugar (which is something you'll find you need to watch out for as well). It also has the advantage of sometimes helping weight loss, and may help girls have more regular menstrual cycles.

Your doctor may choose not to put you on metformin if you have:

➤ Kidney disease
➤ Liver disease
➤ Severe infections
➤ Or if you abuse alcohol

Note: If you take metformin (Glucophage), ask your doctor about going off it temporarily if you have any illness that could cause dehydration. In that case, you may need to start taking insulin or increase your dose if you are already taking insulin. The most common side effect of taking metformin is stomach and intestinal disturbances, but this usually fades in time. Also, you will help this medication work best if you continue to eat healthy and exercise. Simply taking your pills will not do that job for you!

If the pill you are taking does not do the job in controlling your blood sugar, your doctor may add either another oral agent or insulin. Over time, you may need to try even more different pills and combinations to see which ones work best for you. In any case, it is important to know that everyone is different, and that everybody responds differently to treatment. You may find that sometimes several treatments or a combination of treatments will have to be tried before you find the one that works best for you.

The other thing to keep in mind is to try not to be discouraged as you are trying different treatments. It does not mean that your diabetes is getting "worse" just because you need pills or insulin. Sometimes, especially when you have stress in your life, you might need insulin for a while until blood sugar levels improve. When you are stressed, you are more likely not to eat right or exercise. Stress hormones cause blood sugar to rise and a need for more insulin, so it pays to learn how to positively cope with stress. And every teen experiences stress, whether it has to do with doing your homework, getting along with the kids at school, or starring in your class play.

IF YOU NEED TO TAKE INSULIN

As we first found out in Chapter 1, the pancreas is the organ that makes insulin. Back in 1921, when insulin was first discovered, scientists used insulin taken from the pancreases of pigs and cows to give to humans. Today, however, it is made in a lab by a process that makes it just like human insulin. There are different types of insulin, and your doctor will decide which ones might be best for you. The types differ from each other in terms of the length of time it takes them to work.

There are rapid-acting (lispro/Humalog), short-acting (regular), intermediate-acting (NPH lente or glarqine/Lantus), and long-acting (ultralente) insulins. If you need insulin, you may need to learn to mix two types of insulin together for injection.

Insulin also comes in premixed forms, such as 70 percent NPH/ 30 percent regular, for example. Another mixture has 75 percent intermediate-acting/ 25 percent Humalog already mixed. The premixed insulins are convenient and eliminate the need to mix two kinds together, but the disadvantage is that you cannot change the proportions of the dose. Over time some people learn to adjust their insulin based on their food, exercise, and blood sugar numbers, but this is something you do not have the flexibility to do on premixed insulins.

If you do need to take insulin, it's very important that you measure it accurately, so that you don't make mistakes. It becomes even more challenging when you must mix two kinds of insulin together. If you happen to draw up too much or too little insulin, it can cause your blood glucose to be too low or too high. You will also need to inject it into different spots every day. Even if your doctor has asked you to use only your abdomen, you will need to rotate the injections all over the area in order to avoid puffy spots. When you inject your insulin repeatedly in the same spots, a thickening can develop in your tissue under the skin that looks like a lump. Insulin doesn't work well when it is injected into the lumps because it is not absorbed right and then it won't work for you.

Insulin should be kept cool, but should not freeze. Likewise, it should not be exposed to intense heat or direct sunlight. When you travel, especially in hot weather, it is smart to carry your insulin in a cool protective thermos so that it continues to work well for you. The insulin that you are currently using can be kept at room temperature but should be used within a month. After a month, discard the unused insulin and open a new bottle.

There are also devices made that look like a big pen, and that are called *insulin pens*. They are a convenient way to take insulin. The insulin comes in a special cartridge that fits into the "pen" and has a disposable needle. In some types of pens you throw the whole thing away when the insulin is gone, and in others, you just replace the insulin cartridge. They are easy to carry with you in a pocket, backpack, or purse. You will need to change the needle after every use. If you are not familiar with

---

Bottom Line

Whether you take pills or insulin, it is important to take the right doses at the right times.

---

them and you take insulin, you may want to ask your diabetes educator about using a pen.

An insulin pump is another way of getting insulin that many teens (especially those with type 1 diabetes) use for insulin delivery. A pump is a small device, about the size of a pager. Inside is insulin that is pushed in tiny doses through a small tube to a soft needle that you place in your tummy, hip, or leg. You must change the needle and tubing every 2 or 3 days. It gives insulin all of the time, and you program it to give you extra insulin when you eat or snack. Your doctor can tell you if you might be a good candidate for insulin pump therapy. Although the pump has been mostly used for people with type 1 diabetes, there are more and more people with type 2 diabetes who use one.

Maria's and Tyrone's Story

Maria was feeling grouchy. She hadn't slept well in the hospital bed last night. She was hungry. She hadn't gotten her homework done with all of the interruptions, and this morning she had to give herself a shot of insulin, her first. Actually, she was surprised at how well it went. She never thought she'd be able to do it, but she did! It really didn't hurt that much. Even so, she hoped that she would not have to take insulin shots forever. What a pain! She was trying hard to look on the bright side of things, but right now she was having a hard time finding the bright side. What was positive about this whole situation?

Rita said she could have a "pity party." But then Rita had laughed at the whole thing. Although she was a bit surprised that her buddy would find something funny in her misfortune, somehow the laughter felt good. Rita was really a good friend and was coming to learn about diabetes, too. Maria thought that maybe she should be thankful that she didn't have something worse, like her cousin Mike who had leukemia and had just had a bone marrow transplant. She could also be thankful that her parents and Rita were being great. "Wish I could say that about Roberto," she thought. Brothers were so annoying.

Now she and her family had to go to another diabetes education class. They walked into the classroom where they had been yesterday. She stopped in surprise because there sat an African-American guy about her age, wearing sweats and a cap, and an older man. The guy her age was sitting at the table and had his leg propped up on a chair with pillows underneath a cast. Sally introduced Maria to Tyrone and his dad. Sally explained, "I need to go over the same information today with both of you, and since you're around the same age, I thought I'd do it together. Is that okay?" Maria and Tyrone both nodded.

"Why don't you tell each other a little bit about yourselves?"

Maria, in her grouchy state of mind, didn't feel like talking. She glanced across the table at Tyrone and decided he looked friendly. He obviously had come from home, since their coats were flung on a chair. She wondered how old he was. She figured he was about 18. "Actually, he's built!" she thought as she checked out his large frame and wondered if he played football. He had a wide smile, shaved hair, and white teeth. Tyrone briefly told them that he was 17 and a junior at Lebanon High School. He pointed to a cast on his left leg. He said he had broken his leg last week playing basketball, and after his surgery, there was sugar in his urine. He then had to have a test called an oral glucose tolerance test, where he had to drink some disgusting sweet stuff and have his blood glucose measured. The test showed that his blood sugar had gone too high and now here he was. It was bad enough to have *a cast on your leg and be out of football and basketball, and on top of all that, have diabetes. It just wasn't fair.*

Maria listened and felt sorry for him. At least she didn't have to deal with a cast and a sore leg at the same time as diabetes. She told him her story and he shook his head. She suddenly agreed that it wasn't fair that she should have to be here and have diabetes either. Then, from somewhere in the back of her mind, she heard Grandmama's voice in Spanish saying, "Oh, Maria! WhoEVER said that life had to be fair?"

Tyrone told her that the doctor thought he had type 2 diabetes, since his mother, two of his three sisters, and three grandparents all had it. Plus he was a little bit overweight. But since he was athletic and played football and basketball and wrestled, he always thought that it was okay to be heavy.

Sally remarked, "It's a little unusual that we would have two teens with type 2 diabetes here at the same time, but we are seeing a lot more of this disease these days. Okay, well, let's get started."

Step #5: Watch for Signs of Low Blood Sugar

If you take certain pills or insulin to lower your blood sugar, it is very important to understand about blood sugar that becomes *too* low. When food, insulin, and exercise aren't balanced exactly right, blood sugar can go too high or too low.

Whenever you eat or drink, your body signals the pancreas to make insulin so that the food can be used right away. Blood sugar begins to go up as food turns into sugar. But as your body makes insulin and can use the food for energy, the amount of sugar in your blood falls. When your blood sugar drops, your body can make hormones to make more sugar; it's an automatic mechanism that most people never have to think about! Blood glucose levels go up and down all of the time, running somewhere between 70 and 120 mg/dl (3.8–6.6mmoles) but they don't go above 140 mg/dl (10.mmole/l) (and that would be at two hours after eating, when you would expect them to be high because you have all that food in your system.) On the other side of things, if you haven't eaten for over eight hours, your blood sugar should be stable at less than 110 mg/dl (6.1 mmole/l). This is because your body automatically makes *just enough* insulin to meet the needs of all the cells in your body when you are not eating. Mg/dl means milligrams per deciliter. It is a measurement of how much glucose (mg) is in a certain volume of blood (dl). In Canada, Europe, and other places outside of the United States, glucose is measured in millimoles per liter. You can divide a blood glucose in mg/dl by 18 to get the result in mmoles/dl.

However, if you take certain oral agents (pills) to lower blood sugar, or if you take insulin, low blood sugar (hypoglycemia) can be caused by:

- Not eating enough or at all
- A delayed meal or snack
- Too much medication or insulin
- Exercise
- Alcohol

As an example, when you take insulin by injection, you can be prone to having low blood sugar because the insulin can't be shut off in the way it normally is. So the insulin keeps working hard, even if it's no longer needed! Then it is possible to have symptoms of low blood sugar. So when you take certain pills or insulin, you have to eat regularly so that the insulin has something to work on and your blood glucose levels don't drop too low. By timing your food properly, you will be able to balance how your insulin and food work together, with the goal of avoiding both extremely high or extremely low blood sugar levels (see Figure 5).

Low blood sugar is called *hypoglycemia.* Signs of low blood sugar are feeling shaky, sweaty, clammy, hungry, sleepy, irritable, headachy, uncoordinated, or confused. You may notice that you can't concentrate. You may feel dizzy or have a nightmare or sleep restlessly. Some people complain of being cold when

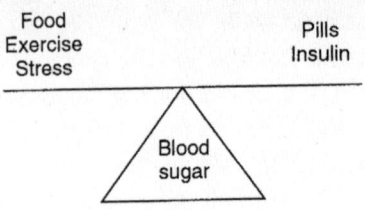

Figure 5: Balancing blood sugar.

blood sugar is low. If you have these symptoms, your body may be telling you that it needs sugar right now. What you must do is to eat or drink something sweet. (Four to six ounces of juice is a great option for treating low blood sugar, or you can chew glucose tablets that are made for just this purpose.)

Signs of Low Blood Glucose

Shaky	Disoriented, confused
Hungry	Uncoordinated
Sweaty	Pale
Irritable	Nightmares, restless sleep
Crying	Tired, sleepy
Can't concentrate	Weak

Signs of Severe Low Blood Glucose

Combative	Irrational	Not able to swallow food or drink
Unconscious	Seizures	

A hormone called *epinephrine* (adrenaline) causes many of the low blood sugar symptoms. It is the same hormone that kicks in when you are stressed or scared. If someone scares you, your heart pounds, you break out in a sweat, your hands get clammy, your knees shake, and you turn pale. These are the effects of epinephrine, which is protective for the body. It has been called the "fright or flight" hormone. Epinephrine prepares you to fight or to run away from danger! When you have low blood sugar, epinephrine gets pumped out.

When you have the signs of low blood sugar, it is important to know whether your feelings are really due to low blood sugar, or for some other reason. Sometimes other things can cause feelings similar to those of being low. For example, you could be hungry because you have low blood sugar, or you could feel hunger simply because you haven't eaten for a while. Or you could feel very tired because you have low blood sugar, or you could be tired because you didn't have enough sleep. You may feel shaky, sweaty, or clammy because you are nervous about a test or a speech. So before you treat yourself for low blood sugar, make sure that you are really low. It is important to find out exactly what your blood sugar number is so that you know how to treat yourself. If you are just normally hungry and then treat yourself thinking that you are low, you might drive high blood sugar even higher.

It is an uncomfortable feeling to have low blood sugar, and people who take insulin can pass out or have a seizure from blood sugar dropping too low. If you experience low blood sugar, treat yourself right away: Eat or drink something that has some sugar in it. Most often, drinking four ounces of juice or taking two glucose tablets will quickly bring blood sugar back to normal. If you don't feel better in 10 minutes, test your blood sugar again and if it is not coming up, have more juice or glucose tablets. Even if you are feeling the symptoms of low blood sugar, as long as you are treating yourself with juice or glucose tablets, your blood sugar levels should eventually return to normal. If for some reason, blood sugar does not rise, or symptoms become worse, call your doctor. Report low blood sugar episodes to your doctor so that adjustments can be made in your plan of care.

Bottom Line

If you have low blood sugar, test your blood first, and then, if you are low, eat glucose tablets or drink juice.

Some people do not sense their low blood sugars very well. It is not completely clear why this is so, although people who have complications from their diabetes are most at risk for this. If you don't know when your blood sugar is dropping, it is a problem because you don't know when to treat yourself with food or sugar. Because you don't realize that you are low, you can pass out. Tell your friends and family that should they ever notice that you are disoriented or confused, or "out of it," you might need to drink or eat sugar. They should know how to help you by knowing what to get, where it is kept, and what to do in case of emergency.

Barry and Julian's Story

Barry is 13 and usually gets home from school around 3:00 P.M. When he went inside and slammed the front door, he hollered for his 15-year-old brother, Julian, as usual. Julian didn't yell anything back, as he always did, but Barry did hear a noise in the kitchen.

Julian was standing there beside the refrigerator with a glass in his hand; nothing was in the glass he was lifting to his mouth. At first Barry thought Jule was just kidding around, so he made a joke, but when Jule didn't respond and kept trying to drink from the empty glass, he suddenly understood. Jule was having another low blood sugar. Barry told Jule to sit at the table and was surprised that Julian actually listened to him. (That never happened!) He found orange juice and poured it into the empty glass, helping Julian to drink it. When Julian chugged the juice, Barry breathed a sigh of relief. Barry found Jule's meter and brought it to him, but Julian didn't pick it up. After a few minutes, Julian looked at Barry and said, "What's going on?" Barry then knew Julian was feeling better and said, "You were low. I think you'd better test your blood. I'm going to call Mom."

Julian remembered then that he didn't take time to eat much lunch that day, and he also had had gym. (Exercise causes muscles to use up sugar faster than usual. Then blood sugar can drop.) The last thing he remembered was getting on the bus to go home. Suddenly he understood why it was important to eat right, especially when he exercised. Thank God for Barry! Who'd have ever thought that the little twerp would know what to do and be able to help? It was a good thing his little brother had gone to the diabetes education classes. When Barry talked to Mom, she said she would call the doctor, because maybe Julian needed less insulin.

TREATING LOW BLOOD SUGAR

When you are feeling "low" the first thing to do is to check your blood. Your diabetes educator might suggest the best meter for you to use, and will show you how it is done on your particular meter. If your blood sugar is less than 70 mg/dl, you should eat or drink something sweet. Most food breaks down into glucose sooner or later. However, some foods that contain sucrose (table sugar) are turned into glucose very quickly. Sucrose and glucose are forms of carbohydrate. Therefore, when you are low, the best thing to do is to eat or drink about 10 to 15 grams of carbohydrate in the form of sugar or glucose, to bring your blood sugar up quickly.

Some sugary foods that work well and contain about 10 to 15 grams of carbohydrate might be:

➤ 4–6 oz. fruit juice
➤ 4–6 oz. regular soda
➤ 2–3 glucose tablets (4 g carb each)
➤ 10 small gumdrops
➤ candy (hard candy such as Life Savers)
➤ others: 2 tbsp. honey, 2 tsp. raisins, 2 tsp. syrup
➤ small tube of decorator gel icing

It is smart to avoid treating low blood sugar with ice cream, desserts, or chocolate. All of these foods contain a lot of fat and calories and will cause you to gain weight. Also, the fat content in these foods delays how quickly the sugar gets into your blood, causing it to take longer for you to feel better. Besides, sometimes when blood sugar is low, it becomes hard to control how much you eat, and you end up eating too much.

ABOUT GLUCAGON

People who are at risk for having a severe low blood sugar episode are those who take insulin. Most people feel symptoms of being low, so it is unlikely that having a severe low blood sugar episode without warning will happen, but it is smart to be prepared. Sometimes a person who is having symptoms ignores them, and does not do anything about it until it is too late for him to treat himself. If your blood sugar drops so low that you are unable to drink or swallow something sweet, you will need an injection of *glucagon*.

Glucagon is a hormone that raises blood sugar. It comes in an injection and should be kept on hand in case you should have a severe low blood sugar episode. Since it should be kept cool, most people store it in the butter shelf of their refrigerator or in a place where it will not freeze. If you take insulin, make sure that a glucagon kit is always available for others to treat you in case of emergency. This means taking it on hikes and when traveling, hunting in the woods, or on overnight trips.

A diabetes nurse educator will show your family how to inject the glucagon in case you should need it. Family members should know where it is kept, and when and how to use it. Your school also should have a glucagon kit on hand in the nurse's office with a doctor's order to give it in case of severe low blood sugar, and there should always be a person assigned to give it to you in case of emergency. (See Medication Management in School.)

As you now know, glucagon is a hormone that should be given to you in case your blood sugar is so low that you are unable to treat yourself by eating, drinking, or swallowing something with sugar in it. A severe low blood sugar episode can cause seizures or unconsciousness. You do not give glucagon to yourself, but will need to show others what to do in case of emergency. The following tips can guide you in what to say. (If you want, photocopy these guidelines and show them to your family, friends, and other individuals.)

Steps for giving glucagon

Glucagon is a hormone that will raise blood sugar. You cannot hurt me by giving me glucagon even if I don't need it.

1. A small vial of glucagon comes in a kit along with a syringe filled with water. Remove the plastic cap from the bottle.
2. Inject the water into the vial, and mix it by rolling or gently shaking the vial until it is clear. It must be mixed right before injecting it, not ahead of time.
3. Withdraw the mixed glucagon into the syringe and inject into the arm, leg, or hip. The needle should go straight in at a 90-degree angle.
4. Give me another injection of glucagon if I am still unresponsive after about 20 minutes. Glucagon can take up to 20 minutes to work.
5. Roll me on my side to prevent choking in case I throw up.
6. Give me something to eat when I wake up.
7. Tell my parents and/my doctor that I needed glucagon.

Maria's and Tyrone's Story

Maria and Tyrone both listened to the lesson on low blood sugar. Tyrone thought about how grateful he was not to be taking insulin at this point. He wondered if he'd ever have to take insulin. He thought he knew what low blood sugar felt like because there were a few times when he was trying to drop a few pounds for football and had quit eating. He remembered being so hungry that he felt shaky and weak. (Dad always said he knew when Tyrone was dieting because he was "crabby!")

Maria, who was now taking insulin, clung on every word Sally was saying. It was scary to think that you could pass out. She asked, "So, if I do what I'm supposed to do, eat right, exercise, take my medicine, and everything, could I still have a severe low blood sugar?"

Sally responded. "That's a really good question, Maria. We would hope not, but there is no guarantee. Think about this for a minute. What makes blood sugar drop? Exercise. Not enough food. Too much insulin. Any one of these things can cause blood sugar to drop too low. If all of them happen at the same time, you are at risk for having a severe low blood sugar. The idea is to prevent that from happening. So as your blood sugar levels fall, your doctor will be cutting your insulin to prevent low blood sugar. If you are exercising you will most likely need to have a snack to compensate for the extra activity. Or if you don't eat enough, your blood sugar may drop unless you learn how to cut back your insulin dose. All of these things together might hit you in a way that could cause your blood sugar to fall pretty quickly. Of course, we would expect that you would feel the symptoms and could treat yourself with glucose tabs or juice. But you should know that sometimes the unexpected happens."

Maria's parents were looking anxious about this new development. Mama began asking Sally if low blood sugar could happen during the night, and if Maria would wake up enough to realize this. "Should I get up and test her blood during the night?" However, Sally said that most of the time that shouldn't be necessary. She recommended that they test blood during the night after a day when Maria's blood sugar was running very low or on nights after she had had a lot of exercise. Otherwise, there wasn't a need to check her sugar during the night. Then Sally got out the glucagon kit and began to show them all about it.

Note: Although it is possible to have times when blood glucose levels run very low, and it is also possible to have episodes of severe low blood glucose, this is not usual. If you are having frequent or severe low blood sugar, tell your doctor or nurse educator so that adjustments can be made in your medication.

Step #6: Eat Healthy and Maintain a Healthy Weight

lifestyle

Managing food has always been a cornerstone of treating diabetes. Before the discovery of insulin, one of the treatments for diabetes was, basically, starvation! Back then, no one knew that there were different types of diabetes, and there were no medications. All that could be done was to limit food. If you had type 2 diabetes and lost weight, you might be okay, at least for a while. If you had type 1 diabetes, though, your life expectancy was probably about a year or two.

Today, if you have type 2 diabetes, following a meal plan and exercising may be the best ways you control your diabetes. You may not need to take medication. The current term for following a prescribed meal plan is *medical nutrition therapy (MNT)*. This plan is balanced to give you consistent calories, carbohydrates, nutrients, and a well-balanced diet. It should allow enough calories to grow and maintain a healthy body weight. If you are overweight, though, it may be a reduced-calorie plan so that over time you can lose weight.

You will meet with a dietitian who will ask you about the types and amounts of foods that you eat, and the times of your meals and snacks. Your plan will be based on how you normally eat, how much you weigh, how active you are, and the type of medication you take. Based on your individual needs, the plan should give you the vitamins, minerals, and nutrients your body needs to be healthy. You will learn about foods that should be the mainstay of your diet, and others that you should eat in limited quantity.

Your dietitian's job is to help you by putting together a meal plan that is both right for you, and that you can live with! If you use your new plan and find that it is not working for you, it may need to be changed a bit. Whatever you do, don't just quit and say, "I can't do it!" Call your dietitian and let her know that you are so hungry before lunch that you end up eating more than

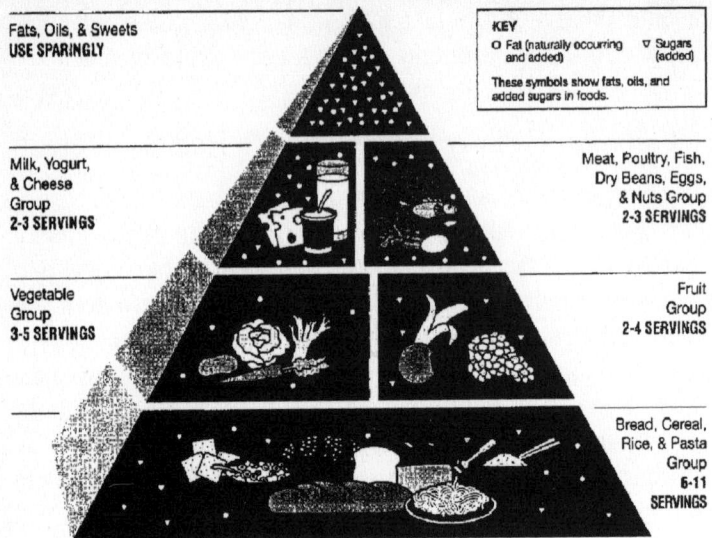

Fats, Oils, & Sweets
USE SPARINGLY

KEY
O Fat (naturally occurring   ▽ Sugars
and added)   (added)
These symbols show fats, oils, and
added sugars in foods.

Milk, Yogurt,
& Cheese
Group
2-3 SERVINGS

Meat, Poultry, Fish,
Dry Beans, Eggs,
& Nuts Group
2-3 SERVINGS

Vegetable
Group
3-5 SERVINGS

Fruit
Group
2-4 SERVINGS

Bread, Cereal,
Rice, & Pasta
Group
6-11
SERVINGS

Figure 6: Food Pyramid Guide: A guide to daily food choices.

your plan calls for, or that the breakfast she has planned for you is too big. That way changes can be made based on *your* needs and preferences, and yet the plan still has a structure to it. Be as consistent as possible with the quantity and types of foods that you eat.

THE BUILDING BLOCKS OF YOUR MEAL PLAN

Because there has been concern that Americans are becoming increasingly overweight, yet can also be malnourished, the U.S. Department of Agriculture designed a Food Pyramid Guide, which gives a guideline to how everyone should be eating (see Figure 6).

At the bottom of the pyramid, or at the base, is the grain group. That group includes bread, cereal, rice, and pasta. A person should eat 6 to 11 servings (a serving is about a half cup, half the size of your fist) of grains every day, and that should be the base of your diet. Next on the pyramid are the fruit and vegetable groupings, each from which you should eat three to five servings daily. Sitting higher on the pyramid are the milk and meat groupings (eat 2 to 3 servings from each), and then the fats, oils, and sweets group. In other words, most of our diet should be grains, fruits, and vegetables, with some meats and milk, and very few fats and sweets. The shape of the pyramid helps you understand which foods you should be eating the most of. This is a healthy way to eat and is especially good for the person who has diabetes. Fats and sweets are not eliminated entirely from the diet, but are a small part of it only; most of our foods should be healthy ones.

People who are overweight often try to lose weight by skipping meals, or not eating much at breakfast or lunch. Sometimes, this plan backfires, however: they end up eating more for dinner and through the evening because they are so hungry. Research has shown that it is better for weight control to eat small meals frequently, rather than to starve and eat a whole lot at one time. Let a dietitian help plan out your meals for you, in a way which works best for you!

THINKING ABOUT WHAT THE FOODS YOU EAT *DO* FOR YOU

It is sensible to think about foods by grouping them by how they fit your needs within a whole day's nutrition. For example, peanut butter and crackers may not be a very smart snack choice for someone who is trying to lose weight, since peanut butter has lots of calories, which can contribute to gaining weight. But peanut butter crackers could be important for a football player to eat before practice to give him sustained energy through practice. A soft-serve ice cream cone may fit very well into the daily plan of someone who ate cereal, skim milk, and fruit for breakfast, a salad for lunch, and grilled chicken and veggies for dinner (in other words, a healthy and balanced diet for the day), and who then craved something sweet. The cone would most likely offer too many additional calories, carbs, and fat, however, for someone who had eggs, hash browns, and sausage for breakfast, a cheeseburger and fries for lunch, and pizza for dinner. Although none of the foods mentioned should be considered "bad" foods, when taken together, in the context of a whole day's food choices, they are too high in fat, cholesterol, and calories, and too low in vitamins and fiber.

WHAT TO DO WHEN YOU GET CRAVINGS

Wouldn't it be great if we all could suddenly turn off our desire for ice cream, burgers, or chocolate? However, the cravings are real, and therefore it is important to make good decisions when you feel such a craving. That doesn't mean that you can't ever have another cream donut or piece of apple pie. But it is important to decide *where, when*, and *how much* to eat if you choose to eat them. In other words, it is important to *plan your food*, rather than eating randomly.

Yes, you may need to dig down deep to dredge up some self-discipline! But one thing to keep in mind is that we are creatures of habit. We like what we like, and we usually eat the way we usually eat. So after you establish some new habits and stick to them for a while, your tastes can change. One teen, after drinking skim milk for six months, decided that he didn't even like the creaminess of whole or 2 percent milk anymore. "It's too rich or something. Makes me feel heavy." Others will tell you that once they've quit eating red meat, for example, they do not even like it when it is served to them later on. You can also acquire tastes for certain foods if you're open-minded and willing to give them a try. Not everyone loves vegetables, for example. Veggies certainly aren't a typical "teen" food, but veggies add vitamins, nutrients, and fiber to a diet, and can be delicious and low-cal if prepared right. By experimenting and tasting different kinds of veggies prepared in different ways, you may find that you can fill up on them and enjoy them.

Bottom Line

There are no junk foods, but there are junk diets. Plan what you eat instead.

PLANNING WHAT TO EAT

Planning your meals and snacks is important. As in anything else you do, success is in the planning! Think about all of the things you make "plans" for. You plan to go out with your friends, you might plan to go to college, you plan a surprise party or plan to go to the prom. The point is that planning is important to *anything* you want to do, and that includes your diabetes care.

When it comes to following a meal plan, for most of us, the planning part is relatively easy. It's the *doing it* part that is hard! However, brilliant military strategists will tell you that success comes from planning and execution. After the planning is done, you will need the help of family and friends to execute your plan. And it is smart to be prepared so that daily changes don't throw you off.

Here are some basic tips that can help you succeed at the meal planning part of your program:

- Have the proper foods and beverages available. (For example, it's hard to drink sugar-free beverages when there is only sugary cola in the house.)
- Know your meal plan! Memorize it so you don't have to look at the written plan of what you're supposed to eat at every meal.
- Weigh and measure your food, at least at first, so that you have a sense of exactly how much you are eating. Once every month or two, it is smart to take a day and weigh and measure your food to keep you on track. It is amazing how a cup of cereal can turn into 3 cups, or how a guesstimated ounce of cheese can become two ounces over time!

- Call ahead to friends and relatives to find out what is being served when you are going over there for dinner or a party. Then you can adjust your food accordingly and/or bring whatever else you might need to fill out your plan. For example, you may need to bring sugar-free soda if you're in doubt as to whether there will be any served.
- Eat small meals frequently so that you do not become overly hungry.
- Decide in the morning what you plan to eat for the day and write down your plan.

Bottom Line

Eating the right foods at the right times is a key to weight loss and good health. Planning is the key to success.

UNDERSTANDING CARBOHYDRATES

Carbohydrates are the body's main source of energy. They are found in fruits, vegetables, and starches such as bread, cereal, milk, rice, potatoes, grains, and pasta. What is important is the total amount of carbohydrates (carbs) that you eat. Almost everything eaten eventually turns into carbohydrate, whether the source is candy, cake, carrots, or mashed potatoes, which then turns into glucose.

When you eat something, it begins to be digested, even in your mouth. Your saliva starts to break down food for digestion. The food goes to your stomach, where it gets broken down even further by digestive juices and is turned into sugar, in the form of glucose. The glucose then travels into the blood and circulates to body cells to provide food for energy.

Because carbohydrates turn into glucose, your blood glucose (sugar) will go *up* after you eat them. That is why your meal plan should include foods with some carbs, but should also limit how much of them you eat. When you eat a big meal with a lot of carbohydrates, your blood sugar can go much too high afterward unless you learn how to balance it with medication or exercise. Besides, just as is the case for everything else you eat, if you overeat, carbs turn into fat. On the other hand, if you *undereat* your carbs and take insulin or certain oral pills, you might be at risk for low blood sugar (see page 32).

It's when you keep the amount of carbs you eat *consistent* from one day to the next that your insulin or pills can balance it to keep blood sugar normal. Your dietitian will help you understand how many carbs should be in your plan.

Types of sugars (all are carbohydrates and found in foods)

Glucose
Fructose—fruit sugar
Lactose—milk sugar
Maltose—malt sugar
Sucrose—table sugar
Dextrose—a simple form of sugar

Bottom Line

Controlling the amount of carbs you eat will smooth out blood glucose, help control weight, and balance medication if you take it.

UNDERSTANDING FATS

Fats provide energy reserve. Like a squirrel putting away an acorn for a rainy day, our body stores energy as fat. During starvation or extreme exercise, the body will break down fat to use for energy. Fats are found in meat, poultry skin, whole milk, butter, margarine, cheese, nuts, and oils. It's hard for your body to turn fat into sugar, and most of the time fat is stored in our body as fat! Fat has little effect on blood glucose levels other than slowing down the digestion of other foods.

Still, it is important to pay attention to the type of fats you eat. High levels of fats in the blood can cause your blood vessels to clog. Fats in the blood are associated with clogged arteries, and diseases of the heart and blood vessels. This does not happen right away, but having a lot of fats in your blood over time can cause problems. You have probably heard about cholesterol, which includes several kinds of fats, and that it's important that your cholesterol not be too high.

Saturated fats are the ones in the diet that raise cholesterol. They are found mostly in animal products, including butter, lard, whole milk, cheese, fatty meats, coconut oil, and palm oil. Healthy choices of oils are corn, safflower, sunflower, soybean, olive, and canola. To know the kinds of fats you are getting in the food you eat, look at food labels.

People, especially teens, may think that cutting the amount of fat in their diet is hard. Well, it *is* a bit hard because of the lifestyle we live, with high-fat foods being served in fast food restaurants and school cafeterias. And Americans do a lot of snacking on high-fat foods. Besides, sometimes you just plain *want* that double burger with fries! But with a little effort, it really isn't all that hard to cut back on the amount of fat you eat. The amount of dietary fat should not be greater than 30 percent of the total calories, with no more than 300 mg of cholesterol consumed daily.

Read labels when you shop, and plan ahead. For example, if you have the choice of having chips (high-fat) or pretzels (fat-free) for a snack, choose the pretzels. If you can eat light yogurt instead of regular, you save fat and calories! Or if you have a real craving for chips, buy the kind that are baked, which have a lower fat content. You might need to help whoever does the shopping and food preparation in your house to understand what you'd like to eat so that foods that work for you and your meal plan are handy.

Here are some tips for you and the cook in your family that

might help you reach your goal of losing weight and eating in a healthy way:

- Trim the fat from meats after cooking.
- Choose low-fat meats (such as fish and chicken) and cheese (mozzarella made from part-skim or light cheese).
- Bake, broil, steam, or poach foods instead of frying them.
- Cook fish or chicken in orange juice or light dressing rather than oil.
- Use a vegetable spray to prevent foods from sticking to pans instead of butter.
- Avoid soaking vegetables in margarine or butter.
- Ask for sauces, such as salad dressings, gravies, etc., to be served on the side. This way you can dip your fork lightly in them for flavor, but can avoid soaking your food in fat.
- Substitute fresh fruit for fattening desserts. Bake an apple with cinnamon and add fat-free whipped topping for a great taste! It has far less fat than apple pie with ice cream.
- Substitute lower-fat for high-fat foods. For example, choose frozen yogurt instead of ice cream, pretzels instead of chips, mozzarella cheese instead of cheddar, sliced turkey instead of salami, etc.
- Eat more fruits and vegetables and less meat and cheese.
- Be assertive in asking how food is prepared when you eat out. Ask if the fish is broiled in butter, if the house salad has dressing already on it, or if the iced tea has sugar in it. If they do, ask the server to change it for you.

Bottom Line

Cutting the fat in your diet will help you control your weight and have a healthy heart.

GETTING STARTED ON YOUR NEW MEAL PLAN

When you start any new program, especially a weight loss program, it may take a few weeks to get used to it. When you have been used to eating a lot, or eating fattening foods and snacks, you may get hungry. Don't let habit tell you to scarf down anything just to be satisfied. It is hard at first to break out of those old patterns, so prepare yourself to be tough for a few days until you get into it. Think about how *good* you will feel to be healthy and have a new, slimmer figure! After a week or so, you will get used to your new way of eating and it should be easier.

That is not to say that you won't ever crave some of your old favorites: You will probably always need to be a bit on guard around tempting foods. Sometimes, once you get started eating those old favorites again, you can't stop! So try to keep as much as possible to the plan you and your team put together. And remember, it does not mean that you won't be ever able again to eat high-fat or sweet foods, just that when you do, you'll need to eat them in *reasonable* portions at the *right* times.

Moderation is one of the keys to success. You will need to know yourself and do what works best for you. The idea is not to feel deprived, binge eat, or snack too heavily. No doubt you will not follow your meal plan perfectly all the time. There are picnics, parties, weddings, school food, and meals in restaurants where it is sometimes hard to be precise about following your plan. Or afterschool activities and possibly sports can throw things off a bit. But try to follow your plan as closely as possible, and use it as a guide to healthy eating and healthy weight. It is your recipe for success! If you follow your guide, it will lead you to weight control, improved blood glucose control, and better levels of fat and cholesterol in your blood. And remember: *When things in your diet are not going perfectly, don't beat yourself up, but try to get back on top of it.*

Here are some tips to help you plan:

• While you are getting started, use measuring cups and spoons and a gram (or ounce) scale to weigh portions. (See page 52 on portion control.)

• Keep food records. You don't need to share them with anyone but your team, but by writing down what you eat, you will have a better awareness of your diet. Write down *everything*, including little bites or "picks" of food, munchies, drinks, and the mayonnaise on your sandwich! Your dietitian then may be able to analyze your records on the computer to see how you are faring with fats, proteins, carbs, vitamins, etc.

• Become a label reader! Reading food labels may not be your favorite reading material, but can be worth the time. It is surprising sometimes what we put into our bodies. You may think that some foods are low in calories or fat, but they're not. The labels tell you how many calories, fats, carbohydrates, cholesterol, and sodium are in each serving. The column "%Daily Value" shows how that food fits into a 2,000-calorie diet (the level most teenage girls and many adults require).

• Know label terms! Just because a label claims that the food is low-fat or non-fat, it doesn't necessarily mean that the food is better for you. Sometimes when the fat is removed, it is replaced with sugar. And some reduced-fat products are not much lower in calories than the regular versions. Besides, when the fat content of a product is lowered, usually the sugar and/or salt content is increased.

Check to see what food labels tell you

• Nonfat or fat-free—½ g of fat or less per serving
• Reduced fat—25% less saturated fat than the standard
• Lean—less than 10 g fat, 4 g saturated fat, and 95 g cholesterol
• Extra lean—less than 5 g of fat, 2 g of saturated fat, and 95 mg cholesterol
• Calorie free—less than 5 calories per serving
• Low calorie—less than 40 calories per serving
• Reduced calorie—at least 25% fewer calories than the standard

- Light or lite—50% fewer calories or 50% less fat
- Cholesterol—a fat found in certain foods, which can lead to clogged arteries
- Low cholesterol—20 mg or less cholesterol and 2 g or less saturated fat
- Cholesterol free—less than 2 mg cholesterol and 2 g or less saturated fat
- High fiber—5 g of fiber or more.

WHAT ABOUT SWEETS?

As mentioned earlier, sweet foods should be at the top of your pyramid (see page 40): you can have them, but they should *not* be the staple of your diet, just an occasional treat. This does not mean that you will never again be able to have a piece of birthday cake. But if and when you do, it should be in the right quantity and at the right times. Your dietitian can help you with "how much and when" guidelines. You might plan to have one or two sweets a week and have them at times when you are being more active. When you do eat them, sit down and enjoy them thoroughly. If you take insulin, don't save sweet desserts for treating a low blood sugar: You probably won't really enjoy it at that time, and it can pack on extra calories.

The biggest, most obvious concern is what happens to your blood sugar when you eat sweets. As mentioned before, sugar is a carbohydrate, and counts in the total carbs you eat. All carbs raise blood sugar, but sweet foods get into your system quickly and therefore can cause a spike in your blood sugar after you eat them. If you eat a sweet dessert at the end of a meal when there is already food in your stomach, however, your blood sugar may not spike up because the food slows the absorption of sugar. And that's a good thing.

How you manage sweets in your diet is also decided by whether or not you take insulin. People who take insulin actually may have an easier time eating something sweet and keeping blood sugar levels normal because they can learn to adjust their insulin for the type of food that they eat. Of course, in this case, just like anyone else who overeats, if you are constantly eating sweets and taking extra insulin to cover it, you will gain weight! And that can make your diabetes harder to control.

If your diabetes is controlled by diet, exercise, or pills, it may be a little more difficult to eat sweets and have normal blood sugar afterward, unless you exercise or eat the sweets with a meal. But let your numbers be your guide. Test your blood sugar two hours after eating sweets and see how high it is. Just remember that eating sweet and fatty desserts regularly will keep your blood sugar levels high and can also promote weight gain.

PORTION DISTORTION

One thing that is contributing to the fattening up of Americans has been the ever-growing size of portions of food. Competition between food companies and people's naturally healthy appetites have contributed to the problem. Fast food places have many sizes of meals: big and bigger! Oh, right: Super Size! Vending machines are switching from 12-ounce cans to 20-ounce bottles, and some convenience store drinks now come in a 64-ounce size. Bakery muffins are sometimes 3 to 4 times the size of the size listed in the USDA nutrition data. America is becoming supersized. Most people tend to eat more than they need or want if the food is set in front of them.

Does the average person need all of these calories? NO! Regular size has gotten bigger. Some places no longer even *sell* small size portions. In general, restaurants have increased the size of their plates in order to accommodate larger portion sizes. Plate sizes have grown from 11 to 14 inches, and some places use platters for dinner plates.

As of this writing, one supersize meal at McDonald's comes close to 2,000 calories, which is close to the *total* calories a teenage girl needs every day, *and* it overspends the fat budget for the day. A Double cheeseburger, Supersize fries, and a 32-ounce soda have 1,800 calories and 85 g of fat.

The thing is, people fall into the big food trap by thinking that for only 39 cents more, they can have all this extra food, which is a "good buy!" It's not a "good buy," however, if it isn't physcially good for you.

Here are some strategies for portion control:

- Downsizing portions at the table might be your easiest strategy for controlling your weight. Cut normal portions in half.
- When eating out with a friend, consider ordering one portion and two plates.
- When eating at fast food restaurants, ask for the nutrition information on their foods. (Most fast rood restaurants have nutritional information for their standard menu in a brochure or flier.) You can make smarter choices when you know the calorie and fat content of the food you order.
- When eating out, eat half and take the rest home for another time.
- Use a luncheon-size plate for dinner and start off with a salad.
- Drink plenty of water!
- Order an appetizer or two instead of an entreé.
- Ask how large the portion sizes are before ordering.
- Divide snacks, sweets, etc. into portion sizes and store in individual zippered bags.
- Buy individually wrapped portions, such as cheese slices.
- Pay attention to how hungry you are. Do you really need the large instead of the medium size?

Size guide:

One serving size is
3 oz of meat, poultry or fish—about the size of a deck of cards
1 small potato—size of computer mouse
¾ cup ready-to-eat cereal—size of tennis ball
1 inch of hot dog or sausage—about 100 calories

Bottom Line

Portion distortion adds unnecessary calories. Take action and don't eat more food than your body needs!

Maria's and Tyrone's Story

Wow! There certainly was a lot to understand! Tyrone adjusted his hat again and wondered how he was going to do this. Although his dad was there and did most of the cooking, he knew how much Dad liked sour cream, steaks, and bacon. He thought of the creamy soups, sausage, and hearty steaks on the grill that Dad made. As if reading his mind, Dad said, "Well, son, this is going to be good for me, too! I sure could stand to lose a few pounds, and the old ticker won't mind, either! Don't worry, you're not going to starve. You know, remember that I told you that a long time ago, I took a summer job on a cruise ship and was a kitchen assistant. Mostly I washed dishes, but I watched the chefs and I learned to make all kinds of vegetables and fruit dishes back then. I never had the money to buy fresh stuff back then, but I think now's the time." Tyrone glanced at his dad and was both thankful and doubtful. "This," he thought, "should be interesting!"

Terri, the dietitian, and Tyrone talked about the way he usually ate: a light breakfast, school lunch, big afterschool snack, and late supper. They put together a plan of food groups and times based on Tyrone's usual day. Terri estimated that he was eating about 3,500 calories a day, and mentioned that during football season he might even lose weight on that amount. Terri commented, "Tyrone, since you don't need a pill or insulin to control your blood sugar at this point, your main goal is not to eat too many carbs at one time, watch your sweets, and cut the amount of fat and calories you eat a bit. You should be able to do this without too big a problem. And all of your sports and athletics will help."

Tyrone was still doubtful. "So what can I have that I like?" Would all the stuff he liked be off-limits?

Dad spoke up. "Tyrone, think about your cup being half full, not half empty! Think about what you CAN have, not what you can't. There are all kinds of foods that you can have that you like—chili and taco salads, baked chicken and mashed potatoes, salads, fruit, corn bread, stuffed peppers, pizza, and homemade bread. You love all that stuff! Besides that, some of those foods that you think you CAN'T have, I'll bet you could have at the right time in the right amounts. Your big thing, boy, is that you are going to have to lay off the sweetened iced tea and regular soda and drink sugar-free instead. That all by itself will help a lot." He turned for confirmation. "Isn't that right?"

Terri nodded and commented, "What your dad said is true, Tyrone."

Maria and Rita then sat quietly while Terri reviewed Maria's meal plan. Terri told them, "It is important for Maria to follow her meal plan very closely because her goals are not only to lose weight but also to balance the insulin she takes. If the food and insulin don't balance, her blood sugar will be too high or too low."

Maria felt angry. She didn't want to do this. In fact, she didn't want any part of it! Tears stung the back of her eyes, and she felt miserable. Rita nudged her in the ribs and whispered, "Come on, Maria, I WANT to learn this. I want to lose weight for summer. This is good for us!"

Maria was glad that Rita was going to stick with it, and with her. At least if Rita watched, too, she wouldn't be sticking Snickers in her face at lunch. And, well, it would be nice to fit into her clothes better, and to not feel fat. Maybe there would be some good in this, too, if she could actually lose weight.

MORE ABOUT HEALTHY EATING

Increase Your Fiber

Fiber comes from plant carbohydrates, which are not completely broken down during digestion. They are found in grains such as whole wheat, rye, corn, oats, and brown rice; dried beans and peas; and all fruits and vegetables. Eating a diet rich in fiber can be good for your general health and also may help with your diabetes control. Here's why:

- Fiber takes up space in your stomach and actually may cause you to eat less because you feel full faster.
- It causes blood glucose levels to rise more slowly after a meal.
- It may help reduce the risk of colon and rectal cancers.
- It adds bulk to your diet and prevents constipation.

So when you have a choice, go for a food that is high in fiber. Here are some easy ways to do this: Choose bran cereal instead of corn flakes, brown instead of white rice, and whole-grain bread instead of refined white bread. Leave the skins on fruits and vegetables (edible ones, that is—skip the banana peel!). Eat fresh fruit rather than drinking fruit juice: An orange has more fiber than OJ, and can make you feel fuller on the same number of calories.

Pass on the Salt

Unless you have high blood pressure, it is probably not urgent that you severely cut back on the amount of salt you eat. But in general, most people have a diet that is high in salt. It is not actually the salt that is the problem, but the sodium that is in the salt. (Sodium chloride is another name for salt.) So if you eat a lot of salt, you take in a lot of sodium. It is the sodium that contributes to high blood pressure and kidney, heart, and blood vessel disease.

Therefore, everyone should be careful about the amount of sodium they eat, and people with diabetes should be even more careful than others. Even if you are a teen who has been healthy and has no problem, it is smart to limit salt to start healthy habits and prevent problems later on. Because people with diabetes are more prone to having heart, kidney, and blood vessel problems, the goal is to prevent high blood pressure in the first place. Cutting down on salt in the diet is part of a healthy eating plan.

Sodium is in many prepared foods, frozen foods, and fast foods. If your diet is big on these foods, you are probably getting more sodium than you need. Don't add extra salt to your food, especially before tasting it.

Bottom Line

Be aware of the amount of salt (sodium) you are eating. Avoid adding extra salt to anything.

Foods Fads and Supplements

Lots of people seem to have their own theories on how to lose weight. Some weight loss programs are healthy, while others are either a waste of money or downright unhealthy. You've probably heard the expression, "It's a fad." The expression usually means a "craze," or something that is popular to do for a short period of time. Hairstyles, dress styles, or attitudes toward food all can be faddish. People follow them because everyone else does. But fads usually fade as quickly as they start. After you quit a fad diet, you regain the weight because the diet doesn't teach you how to eat right and maintain a healthy weight.

Fad foods or fad diets are about what you will or won't eat, which might be based on what other people do. Others might think eating a certain way will make them a better athlete, stronger, healthier, or thinner, or will give them beautiful hair, nails, or skin. Diets such as the "grapefruit diet," the "gelatin diet," "the all-protein diet," "the low-carb diet," or the taking of nutritional supplements to develop muscle may promise to do this.

Unfortunately, most food fads don't do what they're intended to do, and some of them may cause harm along the way. Take a diet that promotes eating a lot of carrots, for example. Raw carrots are generally a food that is considered good for you. A carrot contains fiber, a lot of vitamin A, a little calcium, vitamin C, and carbohydrate. However, if you eat only carrots, as the diet calls for, you miss out on other nutrients that your body needs, such as proteins, other vitamins, micronutrients, and iron. And the coloring that makes carrots orange can permanently discolor your skin (making *it* orange) if you eat enough of them. A carrot is a wonderful, healthy food, but *only* when eaten in reasonable quantities in a well-balanced diet. So if you are thinking about going on a particular diet, first check it out with your dietitian. See charts 1 and 2.

And what about supplements? Many diet supplements are expensive, and some of them are actually *dangerous*. Most of the time, if you eat a healthy diet, you can end up matching on your own the nutrients you can get in an expensive diet supplement, such as protein drinks. But if you have diabetes, you must be very careful about taking protein and sports drinks, as they often contain large amounts of carbohydrates that would need to be taken into account in your meal planning and daily calories.

Creatine is a supplement food that has been highly promoted for athletes. However, its use can be problematic for someone with diabetes because the protein in it can put a strain on the kidneys. So avoid it, because following a normal, healthy meal plan will provide enough protein to meet your needs.

Another product commonly promoted to enhance insulin sensitivity is chromium piccolonate. Although it may have some benefit for people with type 2 diabetes, the benefits may be quite small. If you are thinking about going on a particular diet or using a diet supplement, first check it out with your dietitian. Have you heard the expression "If it seems to good to be true, it probably is?" Unfortunately, everyone wants a quick fix to diabetes, but there are no quick fixes available.

Chart 1. Pros and Cons of Various Weight Loss Methods

Method	Advantages	Disadvantages	Comments
Conventional diets	Safe. Effective at first. Does not require medical supervision. Allows social life that involves eating.	Slower weight loss. Becomes "boring." Does not deal with stress-related eating. May not address need to exercise. Low long-term success rate.	The most common type of intervention.
Aerobic Exercise (walking, jogging, cycling, swimming)	Largest amount of weight loss is in fat. Increased heart fitness and improved muscle tone and appearance. Improves insulin action.	Slow to minimal weight loss, especially in women. Must be done consistently and enough time must be allotted.	Sticking to it is often a problem.
Behavior Modification	Deals with weight loss, maintenance behaviors, and stress related eating. Research supports its effectiveness.	Slow weight loss. Most effective as part of a comprehensive program.	May be related to the effectiveness of a specific therapist.
Pharmacologic (Drug) Therapy	Studies support its effectiveness. Increased rate of weight loss over time.	Most demanding in terms of level of commitment and time. Expensive. Weight may be regained when you stop.	Not clear how long people can safely stay on medication.

Method	Advantages	Disadvantages	Comments
Psychotherapy	May help understanding of the cause of obesity. May be useful if much of the reason for excess weight is emotionally based.	Research does not support psychotherapy alone as an effective weight management technique.	Useful when done in conjunction with structured weight loss program.
Very low calorie diet programs	Rapid weight loss. Little hunger. Safe under medical supervision. Food choices laid out for you.	May lead to metabolic slowdown. Difficulty dealing with normal food selection once the "fast" is over.	Only recommended when under medical supervision. Should be employed only when weight is >50% ideal body weight. Use for limited time only.
Gastric surgery	Rapid weight loss. Most experience early success.	Major medical complications. Does not address psychological problems. Expensive. If eating behaviors do not change, weight can be regained.	Only for morbidly obese who are >200% of ideal body weight or for other medical reasons. Requires follow-up program. May be covered by insurance.

continued

Chart 1. Pros and Cons of Various Weight Loss Methods (*continued*)

Method	Advantages	Disadvantages	Comments
Multimodality programs	Includes food, exercise, behavior modification, and education. Acceptable amounts of weight loss. Deals with psychological factors. Research supports this approach.	Needs major personal commitment. Long-term maintenance required.	Comprehensive approach has much merit. A sensible, if expensive, approach. No guarantees of success.
Pharmacologic and multimodal programs.	Most effective for stress or emotional eaters. Includes food, exercise, and behavior modification. Acceptable amounts of weight loss.	Most demanding approach in terms of level of personal commitment and time. Long term maintenance required. May regain weight after discontinuing medication.	It is not certain how long people can safely stay on medication.

Chart 2. Fad Diets: How they Compare

Eating Plans	Premise	Author	Recommendations	Caloric Guidelines	Low Nutrients	Negative Aspects	Scientific Evidence
Food Pyramid	A healthy lifestyle includes nutrition and physical activity. Includes all food groups.	USDA & Health & Human Service dietitians; reviewed by panel of health experts.	50-60% Carbs. 20-30% Fat 10-20% Protein	1,600-2,800 depending upon whether male or female & activity level.	None, if the pyramid is followed.	None, if the pyramid is followed.	Studies have proven that the most effective weight-loss program balances healthy eating with regular exercise.
Sugar Busters!	No sugar in the diet. Authors say sugar is toxic, causing it to release insulin and store excess sugar as fat.	A corporate CEO and 3 medical doctors.	No firm guidelines. Advises against carbs, espec. simple refined carbs. Focus on protein & fat.	800-1,200	Carbs Vitamins Minerals Fiber	Long-term effects may be increased risk of: heart disease, kidney & liver damage. Short-term effects: fatigue, weakness, irritability.	Testimonial claims support it. Evidence based on opinion, not scientific facts.

continued

Chart 2. Fad Diets: How they Compare (*continued*)

Eating Plans	Premise	Author	Recommendations	Caloric Guidelines	Low Nutrients	Negative Aspects	Scientific Evidence
The Zone	Claims carbs. make you fat. Says most bodies overproduce insulin when we eat carbs. Promotes exercise.	Barry Sears, who has a Ph.D. in bio-chemistry & no formal training in nutrition.	40% carbs 30% protein 30% fat	800-1,200	Carbs Vitamins Minerals Fiber	Takes pleasure out of eating by regarding food as a medicine prescription. Also, fatigue, weakness, irritability.	No scientific proof; supported by testimonials and poorly conducted studies.
Diet Revolution	A throwback to the 70's high protein, low carb diets. Says carbs make you fat.	Dr Atkins is a medical doctor; no formal training in nutrition.	As much meat & fat as you want.	800	Carbs Vitamins Minerals Fiber	May increase risk for heart and kidney disease. Fatigue, weakness & irritability.	It has not been proven scientifically & is supported by testimonials.
Protein Power	High protein, low carb diet; claims the body has no need for carbs; therefore, avoid carbs	Authors Michael & Mary Eades are medical doctors with no formal training in nutrition	30-50% fat 30-45% protein 15-35% carbs.	No guidelines are provided; warnings against <850-1,000 cal/day.	Carbs Vitamins Minerals Fiber	May add stress to kidneys and heart. May increase risk for heart disease.	Claims success through testimonials and book sales.

Eating Plans	Premise	Author	Recommendations	Caloric Guidelines	Low Nutrients	Negative Aspects	Scientific Evidence
Dr. Bob Arnot's Revolutionary Weight Control Program	Claims foods are drugs and make you feel good or bad. Refined carbs are a big factor of weight gain.	Author Bob Arnot is a medical doctor but admits he is not a weight-loss expert.	55-65% carbs 20-25% protein 15-20% fat	No guidelines are provided	Some forms of carbs. Vitamins Minerals	May take a psychological toll as labeling food may make some people who eat a "bad" food feel like a "bad person."	Arnot's theory lacks supporting scientific study.
Eat for your Blood Type	Claims people absorb & react to foods differently depending on blood type 7 ancestors.	Peter D'Adamo: a Naturopathic Physician.	Type O—eat meats; Type A—fruits, veggies & grains; Type B—oat & rice flours, bananas, & prescribed foods; Type AB—tofu, oats & rice.	1,200 or less.	Depending on blood type, whole food groups are eliminated. Vitamins Minerals	By eliminating entire food groups some essential nutrients are deficient or absent.	No scientific or historical evidence for using blood type as an eating guide to lose weight.

Source: Adapted from Wheat Food Council & Washington State Dairy Council, 1999 #DC64.

Bottom Line

Before taking a food supplement or starting a fad diet, talk with your doctor or dietitian.

Another currently popular diet is one that is very low in carbohydrates. Problems with these very low-carb diets are:

➤ Increased risk of heart disease.
➤ Increased risk of cancer.
➤ Poor long-term weight control.
➤ Reduced athletic performance. (Athletes need to carb-load. When you deprive yourself, you're hurting your chances.)
➤ The possibility of kidney stones, gout, high blood pressure, bone loss, and fainting.
➤ Following a very low carbohydrate diet for a long period of time can cause you to feel sick. That's why most people can't stay on a very low-carb diet for very long.

Here are some red flags that may signal questionable diet programs.

➤ Program promises a quick fix
➤ The product comes with lots of warnings
➤ It sounds too good to be true
➤ Selling tactic is based on testimonials from people, but not well-documented research
➤ Statements are refuted by reputable scientific organizations
➤ There are lists of "good" and "bad" foods

Bottom Line

The best way of eating is to eat a moderate amount of a wide variety of foods.

About Dieting

Losing weight seems to be a national obsession these days, but unfortunately a lot of the time, people aren't successful at it. What happens is that people go "on a diet" but don't really change the way they eat. So when the diet is over, they go back to all of the unhealthy practices that caused them to gain weight in the first place. Developing healthy practices does work, and that includes exercise.

Because most teens with type 2 diabetes are overweight, it is very important to lose weight and control eating. You may have tried to lose weight before diabetes. It is hard to lose weight because it is a gradual process. It takes focus, patience, and determination. It takes being a little bit uncomfortable when you are hungry. And it takes discipline! Remember that you didn't gain weight overnight, and you aren't going to lose it overnight, either.

One way to track your progress of weight control over time is to look at your Body Mass Index (BMI). Your BMI is based on your height and weight, and is a percentage of how much you are over or under your ideal body weight. Calculate your BMI, then look at the charts. To figure out your BMI, divide your weight (in pounds) by your height (in inches). Divide that number again by your height (in inches) and multiply by 703. Put a mark on the appropriate graph for you to indicate your BMI, and see if your BMI is above or below the 50th percentile line for your age. If you have trouble doing the calculation, ask a parent, friend, or member of your health care team for help.

A normal range of BMI for children and teens is 15 to 27 kg/m². Recently a teenager's BMI has been associated with how much sugar-sweetened beverages he or she drinks. One study showed that teens who drank sugary beverages every day were most likely to become obese. In other words, drinking high-calorie sugared beverages might cause you to be overweight and have a high body mass index.

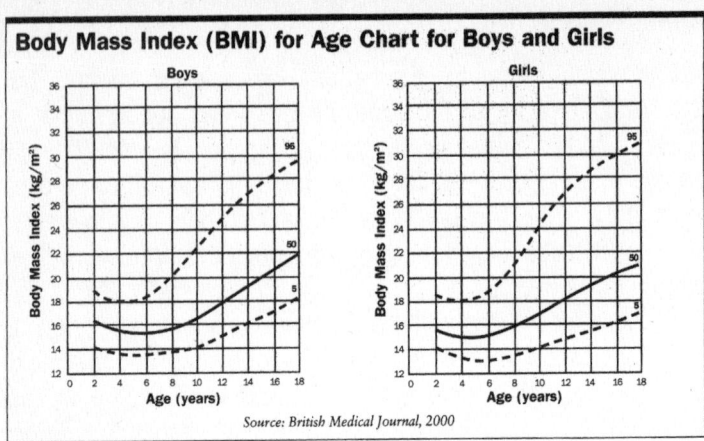

Body Mass Index (BMI) for Age Chart for Boys and Girls

Source: British Medical Journal, 2000

Maria's Story

*Maria and Rita made faces at each other as Terri talked.
They were trying not to be rude, but it was just all so
familiar. They were often teased about how they loved to
eat, and they talked about food a lot! The afterschool
project on Thursdays was always cookie baking, either at
Maria's or Rita's house. They had tried making just about
every imaginable kind of cookie, but of course, half the fun
of making them was eating the batter and fresh-baked
cookies.*

*Maria wondered how much of her extra pounds were
due to cookie batter. She knew that she ate too many
cookies, and had once tried to come up with a diet cookie.
They had left out the shortening, sugar, and salt. What
turned out was so awful that they were still the brunt of*

Bottom Line

The best way to lose weight is to have a healthy lifestyle. Don't
pig out or drink sugary beverages, watch fat, and exercise.

family jokes: "The day Rita and Maria tried to poison us with the baked hockey pucks!"

So they had decided that if it wasn't a "real" cookie, it wasn't worth making. "Now, how am I going to deal with diabetes and cookie baking?" Maria wondered. At the moment, Maria didn't feel at all like giving up cookies.

Then again, perhaps it really wasn't the cookies she valued, Maria realized, as much as the fun she and Rita had together when they were baking

"Well, let's figure out something else to do together!" Rita suggested. "After all, look at us! Look at these legs! Not to mention hips. I don't need all those cookies. Those cookies are going to ruin our shapes! We won't look good in our bathing suits, and we won't fit into our shorts this summer! I'm sick of being fat! This roll here . . ." she said, pinching up her midriff, "is made out of cookie batter!"

Maria started thinking about all of the crazy diets she and Rita had been on together. There were times when they didn't eat breakfast or lunch. Then they'd come home after school and eat more than they would have eaten for either breakfast or lunch anyhow. So that didn't work! Then there was the "only eat fruit" diet, which left Maria unsatisfied but worked until she got diarrhea and Mama was worried about her. After that, she tried the all-protein, no-starch diet where she didn't eat any bread, potatoes, crackers, pasta, or cookies. (But you could eat butter, which she thought was strange.) Anyhow, after about a week of it, she felt tired and then got sick, which ended it.

Maria had been thinking lately that maybe she should save her money to buy some diet supplements at the pharmacy. She saw them advertised on TV all the time. She was interested in hearing what Terri had to say about the supplements because she didn't want to waste her money if they weren't worth it. Rita's mom had tried them and said they were expensive and didn't work that well.

Actually, when she thought about it, Maria realized she had tried everything but giving up cookie baking!

She also thought about her friend Nell, who was dealing with an eating disorder. Maria didn't exactly know what was wrong, but Nell had been missing a lot of school. She hadn't ever been really fat, but just a little bit overweight. She had lost weight and everyone started telling her how great she looked. Maria supposed that had started it, because from then on Nell was different. She seemed tired and didn't call or want to go out anymore. When they'd go to the mall, she'd never try anything on, either. And it seemed that the thinner she got, the fatter she thought she was! For a while she looked great, but then she started looking sick. It was awful, and Maria was worried about her. For a long time, nobody knew she had a problem. Now she was getting treatment and seemed to be doing better, but Maria thought to herself that she would never want to lose weight that way. It must be awful!

Terri was now saying, "There is no magic potion that is going to make you lose weight, at least, lose it in a healthy way. It is hard work to lose weight, but the very best way is to cut your calories and increase your exercise!" Maria started thinking that maybe she could lose weight in a healthy way. Besides, it would feel good to have control of her eating and not let food control her.

Disordered Eating

Sometimes when people want to be thinner and don't control their eating, they are tempted to use bizarre ways to control weight. Probably everyone has either starved or eaten far too much at some point in their life. But when such behaviors continue and are connected with emotions and feelings of self-worth, sometimes an eating disorder can develop. Eating disorders are most common in teenage girls and young women but are not unheard of in men.

One disease, called *bulemia,* is a disease of binging and purging. If you have ever eaten way too much at one time, you might identify with the word "binging." In someone with an eating disorder, however, a binge might include eating huge amounts of food, then throwing up on purpose or taking laxatives to get the food out of their system before it is digested. When a cycle of starving and binging begins, this is bulemia.

Anorexia nervosa is another eating disorder common to teens. It can happen when a distorted perception about one's weight causes deliberate starvation in an effort to lose even more weight. People who have anorexia go to great lengths to hide how thin they are as they become thinner and thinner. Anorexia nervosa occurs mostly in females, and is dangerous in that the starvation can lead to death. When it happens in someone with diabetes, it increases the risks of severe problems.

People who develop eating disorders usually do not recognize or admit that they have a problem and may not do anything about it until others recognize it. And by then it may be very difficult to control the disorder. For example, the disease might start out slowly in an effort to lose a few pounds but slowly become more and more of your focus. It may start, for example, with self-induced vomiting after a big meal once or twice a month, but then progresses to once or twice a week and then to every day. As all the vomiting is embarrassing, the person with bulemia doesn't want anyone to know about it. As time goes on, she becomes obsessed with food and weight loss and feels fat even if she is in actuality wasting away.

If you suspect you are having a problem that could lead to an eating disorder or that you have an eating disorder, you MUST talk to your doctor immediately. Most likely, it will take work with a medical team, your diabetes doctor, psychologist, dietitian, and social worker to get it all sorted out and get you on your way to health.

> ### Bottom Line
>
> Having an eating disorder can be especially dangerous when you have diabetes. Tell your health care professional!

Step #7: Exercise!

There are several important reasons why people with type 2 diabetes should exercise. Let's recall what happens in your body when you have type 2 diabetes: the insulin is not used properly, and therefore glucose cannot get inside the cells. The amount of body fat you have is in proportion to how well insulin works. In other words, the more body fat you have, the harder time insulin has doing its job.

People with type 2 diabetes who are successful at losing a few pounds can improve the way their insulin works. Sometimes even a ten-pound weight loss can make a *huge* difference in how well the body can use insulin.

Another wonderful thing that happens when you exercise: your exercising muscles use more sugar. So when you exercise, you use sugar quickly and the level of glucose in your blood can drop. People who work out really hard or "train" might notice a lowered blood sugar for up to as long as 30 hours after an intense workout. After exercise, blood glucose levels can be much lower for a whole day. You may find that you need to eat more carbohydrates to prevent blood sugar from dropping.

Regularly exercising can lower not only blood sugar, but the amount of fats in your blood. It also cuts your risk of high blood pressure, heart attack, and stroke. It improves the density of your bones, your mood, *and* your shape!

So, being physically fit is both healthy and fun! Most people who develop type 2 diabetes, however, are not very active. Having a sedentary lifestyle means that you are a "couch potato." You may spend a lot of time doing activities that do not move your body across space. Spending a lot of time reading or on the computer, playing Nintendo, and/or watching TV are all popular activities that rob you of the exercise that your body needs to burn calories and be fit.

Some families *are* more sedentary that others. And usually obesity tends to run in families. Part of the reason for this may be that family members share similar genes, but a big part of it also is that people who live together tend to eat similarly and do similar activities. So if you know that your whole family eats fried foods and plops in front of the TV all evening with chips and soda, there is some changing that has to take place. Hopefully, others in your family may be willing to try to change their lifestyle with you. It is very important that you have someone who lives with you to be supportive. In fact, it is as important for the family to make changes as it is for the teen with diabetes! (Besides that, physical activity is much more fun when you can do it with someone.) See if you can be a good example for your family and get everyone *moving*.

The whole issue of weight control is one of energy expenditure. If you take more food into your body than it will use, it gets stored as fat. If you eat the extra portions, you will need to increase exercise accordingly. But remember that it takes a lot of exercise to work off a few hundred calories. You have to walk a mile to burn off 100 calories!

Or think of it this way: It takes 3,600 extra calories over and above what your body usually needs to gain one pound. Whew! That's a *lot* of calories! But you could do that by simply eating 36 extra calories for 100 days! (What's 36 calories? 2 sugar-free Popsicles or one donut hole. To most of us, it feels like nothing.) On the other hand, in order to *lose* 1 pound, you need to cut 3,600 calories by NOT eating food that your body needs to maintain weight, *or* by exercising. So the flip side is that if you eat 36 less calories a day for 100 days than your body needs, you can lose a pound! Putting it that way doesn't sound too hard, and over time it can all add up. The key to making it work is *exercise,* which helps you to use calories and keeps your metabolism burning fuel at a high rate for hours afterward.

Understanding Weight Loss

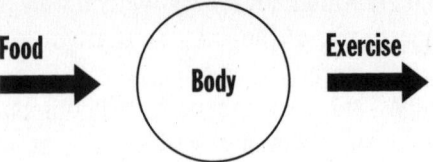

Food and exercise must balance to maintain weight.

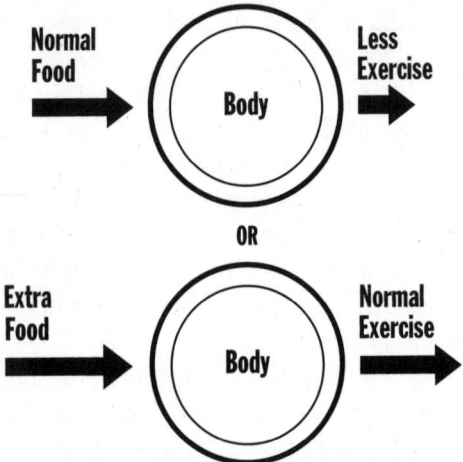

If calories eaten are greater than energy expenditure you will gain weight.

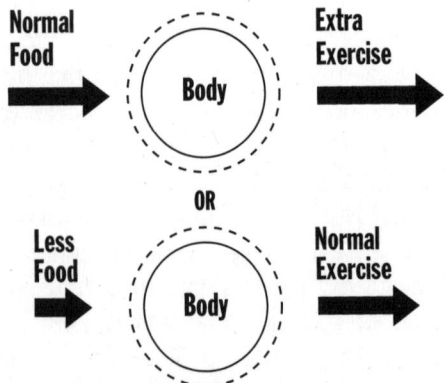

If energy expenditure is greater than calories eaten you will lose weight.

Sports are great ways to get in shape, hang out with friends, and have a blast. Try all kinds of sports until you find one that you think is cool. You may have to shop around for a while until you find one you enjoy doing. You may find that track, wrestling, football, tennis, golf, dancing, and skiing are not your thing but that you really love to bike or dance.

It doesn't really matter what it is that you do as long as it is an activity that you will do *regularly*. The idea is to find something that you really want to do that will get you out there. If it is a drag, you'll be less likely to do it. You might find different activities to do with each family member. Maybe you and your dad will hike in the woods, and your mom will play tennis with you, your sister will swim, and your brother will bike. Anything like this is okay. Whatever works to get moving is great.

Some families will also buy a treadmill or other piece of exercise equipment. This is fine to do as long as you enjoy it and it does not become a chore. Maybe you listen to music, watch TV, or even read while you're walking or on a stationary bike. But if it is a burden to you, most likely you will not continue to do it. If there is a reward in it for you and it is a pleasant, or better yet, *great* experience, you will be more likely to do it. So build the fun into whatever it is you decide to do.

Think about these activities, and see if you could find one or two that are possible for you to do that are also appealing.

➤ Walking
➤ Hiking
➤ Jogging
➤ Rappelling
➤ Swimming (laps, not floating in the water)
➤ Track—cross-country, shot-put, pole vault
➤ Football
➤ Baseball
➤ Basketball
➤ Weight lifting
➤ Crew/rowing
➤ Tennis

➤ Golf
➤ Cycling
➤ Calisthenics
➤ Dance—aerobic, tap, ballet, jazz
➤ Fencing
➤ Gymnastics
➤ Hockey
➤ Karate
➤ Marching band/drill team
➤ Skateboarding
➤ Skating—rollerblading, ice, in-line
➤ Skiing—cross-country, downhill, water
➤ Sledding/tubing
➤ Volleyball

Whatever you decide to do, staying active is key. When you are active, however, if you are taking insulin, you will need to make some adjustments in your insulin or food. Different types of exercise have different effects on blood sugar levels. For example, gymnastics and running cause blood sugar levels to drop more than walking or golf.

WHAT TO KNOW ABOUT EXERCISING WHEN YOU TAKE INSULIN

If you take insulin, you will need to keep an eye on your blood sugar during and after exercise to make sure that it does not drop too low. You will need to ask your team how to make adjustments so that you do not have low blood sugar during or after exercise. Adjustments will be made to your dose of insulin based on:

➤ The kind of insulin you take
➤ The times you take insulin
➤ How tight your usual blood glucose control is
➤ The timing and intensity of the sport
➤ Your usual response to exercise

Bottom Line

Get out there and exercise (and adjust your insulin if necessary)!

Your diabetes educator or doctor will show you how to cut the amount of insulin when you exercise. If something fun arises and you haven't planned on being active and have already taken your full dose of insulin, you will need to cover your exercise with a snack. *Eat two glucose tablets, 4 ounces of fruit juice, and/or four crackers to get through 30 minutes of strenuous exercise.*

Otherwise, if you are not on any medication to treat your diabetes, you will not be prone to having a low blood sugar episode with exercise. Still, it can happen with some of the oral medications. Your diabetes educator should tell you if the medication that you are on could cause blood sugar to fall with exercise.

Tyrone's and Maria's Story

Tyrone listened to Sally talk about being a couch potato. He felt confused. That wasn't him at all! He was always active and doing something. "I do like to eat and I've always been big. But I've NEVER been a couch potato. So how come I have diabetes?"

Sally explained, "Most of the time people are inactive, but type 2 diabetes can also occur in people who are not overweight and are not sedentary. Sometimes periods of stress can cause type 2 diabetes to ebb and flow. With a strong family history of diabetes and being overweight, the stress of your surgery and inactivity may have tipped the balance for you." Sally continued to say that if Tyrone lost some weight, didn't eat a lot of sweets, and stayed active, there was a good possibility that his blood sugar could actually return to normal. But if another stress or weight gain came along, high blood sugar could be a problem again. For now, though, it looked as though the best treatments for Tyrone's diabetes were diet and exercise, and the exercise part would be a challenge until his leg healed.

Maria, on the other hand, listened and felt more and more like the couch potato. She really didn't do much in the way of exercise. Mama used to tease her about not wanting to sweat. It was true. She thought about how she always hated to get out of breath and to sweat. She always looked for excuses not to have to take gym in school. Her activities were Key Club, her church youth group, and voice lessons. She loved to sing and wondered if that counted. She at least was using some muscles when she sang, and while she was singing at least she didn't eat! She and Rita studied the list of activities Terri gave to them. Rita offered, "How about jumping rope? That's not on there."

"That would work . . . Although I don't have a jump rope."

"Well, what do you want to do?"

"I wouldn't mind walking after school. Want to walk instead of making cookies?"

"Yeah!"

While Maria wasn't thrilled at the idea of exercising, the weather was nice now and if Rita would go with her, it might be okay. "We could walk down the to the dairy and get a frozen ice . . . Oh, forget it! Guess that wouldn't work. We could walk to the mini mart and go see that blond guy I have a crush on!" Maria smiled as Rita looked disgusted. "Okay. I know! We could walk to the park. How far is it to the park, Papa?"

"About a mile."

"Okay, so if we walked to the park and back that would be two miles a day. Wish I had a dog . . ." She smiled engagingly at Mama and Papa, who ignored the plug. "And in the summer, we can walk to the pool and back."

Rita continued, "Do you remember Patty, who used to live in that house on the corner? She used to be really fat in high school. I ran into her last week at the mall and I didn't even recognize her. She's modeling now. Go figure! She said she started walking in college, then started running and now does five miles a day. She looks really awesome!"

STEPPING FORWARD

The first steps for taking care of your diabetes have been outlined in this chapter, beginning with your knowledge about diabetes, finding a health care team, monitoring your blood sugar, taking your medication, treating low blood sugar, eating in a healthy way, maintaining a healthy weight, and exercising. As you learn to live with diabetes, you will find that you must achieve a balance among the amount and types of food you eat, exercise, and medication to keep blood sugar levels in line. Following a meal plan and exercising are important in order to achieve a healthy weight so that blood sugar levels can be as normal a possible. By following these seven steps, you are on your way to managing your diabetes in the best possible way.

3

Taking Charge

Let's face it: Most of the time, you have a pretty good idea what you *should* do to maintain your health. You know you should brush and floss your teeth, bathe regularly, visit the doctor and the dentist for checkups, eat healthy foods, get enough sleep, and exercise. The hard part is actually doing it.

When you have diabetes, you have a whole other bunch of "shoulds" to do. You should follow a meal plan, test your blood sugar, keep records, exercise, and possibly take pills or insulin. If only we all could do the things that we should!

Having a chronic disease is hard for anyone. A *chronic* disease is one that doesn't go away. For example, if you have a cold, the flu, or chicken pox, in time the problem will go away. You may need antibiotics or other medications, but the illness is usually short-lived. When you have a chronic illness, however, it does not go away. Many chronic illnesses are easily treated but not cured. For example, sometimes you can take a medication that treats it without any other problem. Other chronic illnesses show effects on the body and in time have negative effects on the body. Diabetes is one of those. Over time, high blood sugar can cause damage to your body such as damage to the tiny blood vessels in your eyes, kidneys, or feet (we'll hear more about this in Chapter 4).

In this chapter I'm going to offer some advice to keep in mind that will help you to gain control of your diabetes despite the fact that it's hard.

Tip #1 for Better Control: Learn as Much as You Can

Make it your mission to learn as much as you can about diabetes and how to control it. Don't be like the ostrich that sticks his head in the sand when he's scared! Diabetes is not going to go away, and the more you know how to deal with it, the better. When you don't take care of diabetes, it takes care of you. (You get the bear or the bear gets you!) It's like it's just lurking, waiting for an opportunity to take control. One teen described diabetes as the "dark shadow, always in the background waiting to pounce." In order to beat the shadow, you must know your enemy.

Now, you may not want to call diabetes an enemy, since you have to live with it every day, but in some ways it is. So be a sponge and soak up as much diabetes information as you can hold! The more you know about diabetes, the better you will be able to handle problems when they crop up. You will then be able to make good decisions about your care.

Learn about diabetes from:

- Your diabetes educator and medical team
- The American Diabetes Association
- Books or magazines about diabetes
- Diabetes support groups
- Camp

Bottom Line

Control diabetes so that it doesn't control you!

Tip #2 for Better Control: Teach Others about It

You will also need to teach others about diabetes. Many people have a poor understanding of diabetes care. Friends and members of your own family may have some goofy beliefs that you will need to straighten out. Sometimes people have been misinformed, or they have certain cultural or family beliefs that are very strong. Usually they know someone with diabetes and make generalizations about what should happen based on what that person does.

So the first rule is: Don't assume these people are good informants! When there is a problem, many people are full of advice. It's okay to consider what others tell you with good intentions, but make sure that you run it by your medical team if the information is different than what you have been taught.

Have people encouraged you to eat, saying, "Oh, just a little piece won't hurt"? Well, lots of little pieces can make for one big hurt, and somehow you will have to kindly and tactfully tell well-meaning Aunt Sophie that encouragement to eat things you shouldn't is not being helpful. You can take control by showing her what you would like her to do. It may be that she wants to help but just doesn't know how. So perhaps you can teach her. For example, maybe you could say something like, "You know, Aunt Sophie, that I love your apple pie, but I really can't eat it. It has a lot of fat in the crust and there is too much sugar in the apples, and that will make my blood sugar go up. Next time, I wonder if you would make a little apple pie just for me with Nutrasweet and very little crust." She might be pleased she could do that for you.

Bottom Line

Learn as much as you can, and teach others!

Tip #3 for Better Control: Look for Patterns

The blood glucose numbers that you get are your tools to keep yourself on track. Just like a carpenter can't build a bookshelf without the tools of a saw, hammer, and nails, it is difficult to be in good control of blood sugar levels without the use of your blood sugar numbers. Sometimes your blood sugar numbers might be within your target. Yet even though you want them to be in your target range, it is also helpful to try to "catch" some when they are not in your target range. Many ostriches do not like to do that (it's that "head in the sand" approach again) because it means something is not exactly right and they don't want to be reminded of that.

But sometimes what you don't know *can* hurt you. So be smart and take a hard look at what your blood sugar numbers look like. Even if you know you ate something that might have caused them to be high, if you are getting numbers that are out of your target range, something needs to be adjusted. One trick that is very helpful is to watch for patterns in your blood glucose control. You may notice that your blood sugar seems to be in your target range at breakfast, but is running over 300 in the evening. That is a pattern, and you should tell your doctor so that an adjustment can be made. Or maybe you notice other patterns with the foods you eat. For example, maybe you notice that your blood sugar runs high after you eat pizza. Or maybe you notice that your blood sugar runs normal on the days that you have oatmeal for breakfast instead of the usual raisin bran. These are all patterns that can be useful in trying to manage your blood sugar. There are also the patterns that you notice if you go off your meal plan and eat sweets. Then you might notice that your blood sugar levels are quite high, or that you are thirsty and having to urinate a lot. These observations are the first step in being able to solve diabetes problems. Talk to your doctor or diabetes educator about the patterns you observe. See the following chart for examples of different patterns that you might see.

Bottom Line

Pay attention to patterns of highs and lows.

Test before and after meals to find out food's effect on your blood glucose.

Name: Sam

Week of: 1–7

Day	Breakfast			Lunch			Dinner			Bedtime		Other/Snack		Comments
	Pre / Post	Carbs	Insulin	Pre / Post	Carbs	Insulin	Pre / Post	Carbs	Insulin		Carbs	Insulin	Carbs / Insulin	Diet, exercise, ketones, illness, stress
M	86		/	124		/	*203		/	97		/	/	*Football practice
T	111		/	189		/	240		/	72		/	/	
W	76		/	100		/	*367		/	86		/	/	*Football practice
T	122		/	94		/	199		/	97		/	/	
F	118		/	136		/	*211		/	111		/	/	*Football practice
S			/			/			/			/	/	
S			/			/			/			/	/	
Avg.	134													

Within Target _____

Above Target   6

Below Target

Pattern: High at Dinner on football days

Name: Liz

Week of: 8–14

Day	Breakfast		Lunch		Dinner		Bedtime	Other/Snack	Comments
	Pre/Post	Carbs/Insulin	Pre/Post	Carbs/Insulin	Pre/Post	Carbs/Insulin	Carbs/Insulin	Carbs/Insulin	Diet, exercise, ketones, illness, stress
M		214 /	Gym	69 /		148 /	92 /	/	Gym
T		193 /		70 /		168 /	111 /	/	
W		183 /	Gym	90 /		124 /	189 /	/	Gym 10 a.m.
T		234 /		102 /		175 /	69 /	/	
F		189 /		79 /	Band	99 /	98 /	/	Band
S		177 /		111 /		*256 /	123 /	/	*Party-out to dinner
S		181 /		138 /		149 /	63 /	/	
Avg.									

Within Target _____   # Above Target _____   # Below Target _____

Pattern: high at breakfast and dinner

Tyrone's and Maria's Story

Tyrone's mind took off, thinking about sports in general, and football in particular. (Of course, that was nothing new. He was always thinking about different plays. He could conjure up almost a whole game of plays in his mind.) In the middle of these thoughts, with Sally talking away, he began to wonder exactly what diabetes was going to mean for his football potential. He had questions. "What if Coach doesn't play me as much because I have both a broken leg and diabetes?" "What if my sugar keeps me down?" "What if I can't get a scholarship because I have diabetes?" Then, even worse, his friend Jerome had told him yesterday that he couldn't be in the military if he had diabetes. Tyrone really hadn't thought about the military because he was bent on getting an athletic scholarship, but sometimes he dreamed of flying a military plane or being a Marine. It was just an option that he always thought he had if the scholarship thing didn't work out. Now what? Maybe his plans would be all messed up. His mind came back to attention when he heard Sally talking about famous people who had diabetes. Some of them were athletes who had diabetes that he really admired, like Wade Wilson, Jackie Robinson, pitcher Jim "Catfish" Hunter, Ty Cobb, NFL football player Jonathan Hayes, and Gary Hall, who recently won an Olympic gold medal in swimming.

At the same time, Maria was also thinking about her future. Maria remembered seeing something recently on the news about the hazards of diabetes and pregnancy. Maria wondered if she'd ever have a boyfriend, and if she found one, if diabetes would make a difference. Of course, the way things were right now, Papa was so strict it might never happen anyway! And she thought about being overweight. Many of the Latino women in her part of town were overweight, but most of the girls her age weren't. She wondered if diabetes would get in the way of her wanting to be a nurse, or getting married, or having a family someday. Sally assured her again that she could do almost anything she wanted with her life, except for being in the military. Then, when she heard the list of famous people who have diabetes, she realized that it hadn't gotten in their way; why should it get in hers?

Some Famous People with Diabetes

Halle Berry—actress
Elvis Presley
Jackie Robinson—first African American in Major League Baseball
Carol Channing—actress and vocalist
Nicole Johnson—Miss America 1999
George Lucas—director of *Star Wars*
Thomas Edison—inventor
Johnny Cash—eight-time Grammy Award winner
George C. Scott—actor and Academy Award winner
Jim "Catfish" Hunter—baseball pitcher in the National Hall of Fame
Ella Fitzgerald—jazz singer with 14 Grammy Awards
Sugar Ray Robinson—boxer
Patti LaBelle—singer
Curtis Mayfield—singer ("Superfly")
Arthur Ashe—Wimbledon tennis champion
James Cagney—actor
Nell Carter—actress and singer
Ernest Hemingway—author
Gary Hall—Olympic gold medalist in swimming
Bobby Clarke—hockey superstar
Mama Cass—singer from the Mamas and the Papas
Jerry Mathers—actor, *Leave It to Beaver*
Mario Puzo—author, *The Godfather*
Jerry Garcia—lead singer of The Grateful Dead
Brett Michaels—singer from the band Poison
Ty Cobb—baseball legend
Howard Hughes—billionaire
Mary Tyler Moore—actress

Tip #4 for Better Control: Play the Hand You've been Dealt

Sometimes it can be discouraging to think that you will have to do diabetes tasks for the rest of your life. Sometimes life gets in the way and you can't keep up with everything. Sometimes it's hard to make yourself do the things that you need to do and you just feel burned out on it all. You may feel as though it is just not fair! It's okay to feel like this. But if you haven't already learned that life isn't always fair, now is as good a time as any to learn that lesson. You could rant and rave and kick the wall, have temper tantrums about it, or become depressed. But the bottom line is that you have diabetes and even though it is understandable that you would have feelings of anger or frustration, all the denial in the world is not going to take it away. You have to play the hand you're dealt, do what you need to do, and move on.

You did not cause your diabetes. You do not deserve it. But now the question is, What are you going to *do* about it? You can spend a lot of time and energy beating yourself or somebody else up, sulking, or being mad. But think about it: You were given certain qualities at birth: your height, skin, teeth, hair, and eye color. Unfortunately, a diabetes risk also comes with the package. You can't change some things, so it is best to pick yourself up, dust yourself off, and get on with life. Get a grip on it and move on.

Bottom Line

Feeling sorry for yourself gets you nowhere. Pick yourself up and move on!

Tip #5 for Better Control: Unglue Yourself

Psychologist Richard Rubin calls any barriers that come up "sticking points." It's kind of like someone putting glue on the middle of a slide. You're sliding nice and smooth and then you hit a snag that makes you get stuck. Sticking points hold you back from doing what you need to do for yourself: they prevent you from moving forward. When you have diabetes, it's smart to try to take some time to figure out why you get stuck, where you stick, and how to get yourself moving again.

For example, what gets in the way of taking the best care of yourself that you can? Maybe it is changing your choice of which door you walk in after school so that you don't have to walk past the fridge. That way, you won't be tempted to eat things that you shouldn't eat. Or another strategy might be to have your snack planned and ready so that when you walk in the door after school, you won't have to spend time looking for and eating not-so-healthy snacks. Or maybe you can start keeping your running shoes in a place that reminds you that they are waiting to be used. Perhaps you decide to put your meter on top of the cereal box so that you have to pick it up to eat breakfast, making sure that you test.

Everyone has some things that hold them back from doing what they want to do or should do. Most teens and adults alike have problems in certain areas. Some folks have no problem testing their blood sugar, but can't seem to work the meal plan. Others might take their medication exactly right, but let their exercise program die. Identify as specifically as possible your own sticking points. Then you need to figure out how to unstick your-self! After all, taking care of yourself, preserving your health, and enjoying what you do are the best gifts you can give yourself or anyone who cares about you.

So start thinking about ways to problem-solve yourself to a solution. For example, maybe you do well all day long and then, after dinner, go crazy eating things that are not on your meal plan. Maybe that is a time when you're bored, or tired, or feel like snacking while you do homework or watch TV, so you start nibbling on chips, ice cream, crackers, or candy. If you know that is your weak time, try to find ways to guard against it. Fill that time with new activities, talk on the phone, nap; whatever it takes! Eventually your new behavior will become a habit, just like your old behaviors.

Let's go over how to problem-solve your way to a solution, by ungluing yourself from your sticking points.

The problem is:	*that in the evening I overeat.*
The sticking points are:	*I am bored.*
	I am tired.
	My guard is down.
	I'm hungry.
	Food is in my face.
	My brother is eating.
The Solution:	*Get all tempting food out of the house.*
	Ask my brother not to eat in front of me.
	Talk to my parents so they can help me.
	Plan some snacks that I can have in the evening.
	Make a rule that there will be no eating during homework or watching television.

You get the idea. Some of the solutions may not be easy, or you may need to get the help of someone such as your parents, doctor, counselor, or diabetes educator. At least you are aware of the problem, and that is half the battle. Once you have defined the problem, you are half done solving it! Once you confront problems, you realize you have options to solve them. You begin to feel in control of yourself and the things that happen to you.

Bottom Line

Know your sticking points, and then problem-solve to unglue yourself.

Tip #6 for Better Control: Enjoy Life

Don't let diabetes keep you from doing the things you want to do. Yes, taking care of diabetes requires time, energy, and focus. The goal is to try to fit diabetes into your life and not have your life revolve around diabetes. Your diabetes care should become part of your routine so that you don't have to think about it. It is a high priority, but it is not healthy to have diabetes be the center of your life. Once you learn to fit diabetes into your life, it should not get in the way of activities or things that you want to do. People who do well managing their diabetes seem to accept that they have diabetes and quietly fit fun things into their life without making it a big deal at all. They just do it, fitting it all in without much fuss.

Bottom Line

Fit diabetes care into your life in the easiest way possible.

Tip #7 for Better Control: Have a Positive Outlook

When misfortune hits, such as having an illness or disease, it is hard to find anything positive about the situation. Having a positive outlook doesn't mean that you don't recognize the problem or that you are in denial. It means that you are willing to accept the things in life that you can't change. Some people can deal with what life dishes out better than others. Ever heard the expression, "When life deals out lemons, make lemonade?" You may have heard a similar expression about your cup being half full or half empty. (In other words, count your blessings and think of your life as being half full.) What about "Every cloud has a silver lining?" Or the serenity prayer, asking God to "grant me the ability to change the things I can change, accept the things I cannot change, and the wisdom to know the difference"? There are many expressions and sayings out there to give you hope. Your outlook depends on how you look at life. For example, although following a meal plan is not exactly fun, one benefit is that you will eat healthier and maintain a healthier body weight than if you *don't* follow it. Your whole family may be healthier if they, too, start eating healthy foods. Although exercising is sometimes hard to get out there and do, it may help high blood pressure and weight control. Appreciate the positives that come out of a situation.

Although having diabetes is a serious problem, it is a disease where you can be healthy and feel well, if you take care of yourself. The good news is that diabetes can be *managed.*

Also, the structure of life with diabetes can teach you discipline, which can carry over into other parts of your life, such as school performance, athletic performance, or playing an instrument. Having diabetes can also give you an appreciation of your health and increased motivation to keep it good. Nobody wants to be sick! Sometimes, however, it just seems too hard to do what needs to be done. But if you do go down that slippery slope, you will land at the bottom in a wipeout. (After all, the less you do for your diabetes care, the worse you feel and the more complications you get.)

Bottom Line

"It is not so much what happens to us in life that matters but the outlook we take toward what happens."—Charles Woodson (football player)

Tip #8 for Better Control: Be Patient with Yourself

As a student, you're probably busy and feel that diabetes is definitely not your top priority. But try to take small steps in the right direction. Remember that diabetes control doesn't happen overnight, and that you will not be perfect at it every day, but that taking care of yourself now will give you better chances for a healthy, happy future.

It is hard to do or not do something today because it could

hurt you in some unknown way in 10 or 15 years. That's pretty tough. If you are like most people, you want what you want right now! When Mom reminds you to test your blood sugar, you might respond, "Why does it matter whether I test or not?" or "I already know that my blood sugar is high because I just ate pretzels," or "I don't want not to eat when I'm hungry," or "Who cares?" or "I don't have time." But keep thinking of the *forest*, not the trees. Think of the marathon, and not the sprint. Think of the big picture. It is doing reasonably well, not perfectly, over the long haul that is important. Try to just do it and not sweat the small stuff. Your future is in your hands.

Think of it this way: from the time you were born, your parents have done the best job they could to raise and protect you. What do you suppose all of those curfews, time-outs, rewards for good grades, having to go to church, eating your vegetables, not speaking to strangers, and other rules your parents make are about? Parents set rules because they love you and want you to grow up to be safe, healthy, happy, and successful. You can test the rules, bend the rules, resist the consequences, and skirt the issues; *or* you can abide by the rules because you know that they are in your best interest for the long haul. It's all about *choices*.

Bottom Line

Choose to be healthy; do it for yourself.

Tip #9 for Better Control: Learn from your Choices

You can choose to study and do your homework, or not. If you don't, you pay the consequences by doing poorly in school, and perhaps being grounded at home. Then maybe you won't be able to go to the school you want, or get the job you want. Or maybe you won't even graduate! People who have long-range vision can see where they want to go and the path that will take them there. Good students might do well in school because they want to be a pilot, a teacher, or engineer, or have a career one day that demands that they do well. The result of the hard work is that it leads to success. Sometimes you don't even know that until you have proven to yourself that you can work for something and achieve it. It takes discipline!

Maybe you aren't the student type, but it doesn't matter because whatever you want to do with your life, whether it is to get a job, raise children, or go to school, you will need some discipline to get up in the morning and do what you need to do.

Being a teen means that sometimes you might do things that older and wiser people think are risky, thoughtless, or stupid. It is normal and natural for you to want to experiment with risky behaviors. But that doesn't mean that those behaviors are either smart or healthy. You may not understand the consequences of the things you do, or more likely, you may think you don't care what happens. Ask some friends if they ever thought they wouldn't care about the consequences of something they did and if it turned out that, in fact, they did care. The answer usually is yes. Or you may just think that nothing bad will ever happen!

Some teens do things just to see how much they can get away with. You may push all sorts of things to the limit as you make choices in life. You choose who you'll hang out with, the kinds of people who attract you, what limits you set on your behavior, and how hard to work or study, among other things. It is a time of finding out who you are and what you are about. The choices *are* yours to make. You may not always make the smartest choices, but learn from your mistakes and move on.

Tip #10 for Better Control: Start Acting in New Ways

Experts have shown that people go through a period of readiness before they start any new behavior. The amount of time it takes to get there, however, can depend on how many barriers (or sticking points) you hit on your way, and how much support you have to jump over the barriers. We seem to have a little switch in our brains that needs to get turned from "off" to "on" before we will do something.

Experts also know that any new behavior won't happen unless it is important to you. Think about what it takes to click the "I'm in control" switch in your brain from "off" to "on." It would be a good bet that if something is extremely important to you, you will find a way to make it happen. See what you can do to make it important to you to take good care of your diabetes.

Here are things other teens have done that they say helped and motivated them:

➤ Put together a support system. Include people from all of your circles of friends: your best friend, your gym partner, a favorite aunt, your clergyman, band leader, athletic coach, diabetes educator, teacher, etc. These should be people you can talk to and who will give you a "high five!" when you need some inspiration.

➤ Communicate well with your heath care professional. That person is on your side, wanting you to do the best you can do with your diabetes, and is there to help. Whether it is a team of people or one person, find someone who is willing to listen to your concerns, answer your questions, and take the time to make sure you know how to manage your diabetes. The responsibility to make the call is yours.

➤ Go to diabetes support groups organized by your hospital or organizations like the American Diabetes Association. There you will learn you are not alone in dealing with your problems. (See Chapter 7 for more information.)

➤ Go to diabetes camp! It is fun and is a good way to make friends. When you are with others who have similar problems, you realize that you are not alone with your problems. If you are too old to be a camper, you might inquire about becoming a counselor-in-training. Camp counseling is hard but fun work; it helps you learn responsibility and looks great on college applications.

➤ Decide to make the best of it. You can't fix it, so just deal with it.

➤ Keep on trying. Having an all-or-nothing approach doesn't get you anywhere. Just keep plugging away.

➤ Find something bigger than yourself to believe in. Pray, listen to music, volunteer your time, or baby-sit a youngster with diabetes: it gets your mind off yourself.

➤ Close your eyes and see yourself as thin, healthy, active, and in good control of your diabetes. This technique is called "visualization," and works because we all tend to go the direction that we see ourselves going. We meet our own expectations.

➤ Avoid negative people who make you feel sad or bad about yourself.

➤ Make sure you have the right supplies available. If you don't have the stuff (testing supplies, right kinds of food, etc.) with you, obviously, you can't use them!

➤ If you find yourself slacking off, ask someone to get on your case until you get moving again.

➤ Figure out ways to remind yourself to do stuff, such as putting Post-it notes on your mirrors or your computer. Or make your new behavior a habit, like getting up in the morning and testing first thing, before you do anything else.

Tyrone's and Maria's Story

It was time to quit for the day, and Tyrone and Maria walked out of the classroom. Maria had a headache and still was feeling, as Roberto would say, "punko." Tyrone seemed to have energy, but he carefully guarded his leg as he placed his crutches around the chairs and wastebasket. He said to Maria, "Well, good-bye. Stay cool." Maria was about to respond by saying that she hoped to see him quarterbacking the Cowboys someday but Sally caught up to them, saying "Oh, wait! No good-byes yet. There is still a lot to learn and we haven't covered it all yet. There is more to go over, although you know the basics. I'll see you both back here tomorrow. Same time, same place! Is that okay with everyone?" Maria and Tyrone looked at their parents for confirmation. They were all tired but knew this was important. They'd be there.

4

Preventing Complications

When diabetes is not well controlled, in time the effects of having continuous high blood sugar levels can damage the tiniest vessels in the body. The damage to the little vessels causes them to leak and not perform well. When this happens, it is called a complication of diabetes, and it can be serious.

Maybe you have heard of some of the problems that people with diabetes get. The damage to the vessels can affect eyes, nerves, heart, blood vessels, and kidneys. If the leaky vessels are in the back of your eyes, you might develop eye problems, or if the leaky vessels are in the kidney, you get kidney problems. When the nerves and vessels in your legs are affected, you might develop circulation problems in your legs or feet. When the nerves become damaged by high blood sugar, you might not be able to feel your feet or have tingling and pain. When the nerves to your stomach are affected, you may not digest food properly. When the nerves to your sex organs become damaged, if you are a male, you may not be able to have an erection, and may become impotent.

These complications sound scary, and should be enough to motivate anyone to take good care of their blood sugar. Many people, however, don't heed the warnings and believe nothing bad will happen to them. That's not a wise way of thinking! But the good news is that these problems don't *have* to happen. You can do something to prevent or delay them. That something is that you can learn what to do to take control of your diabetes, and do it.

Although taking charge of your blood sugar and sticking with your program is not easy to do, it can be done. Many teens and adults alike do very well taking control of their diabetes. You may need to be tough with yourself until you get on track, and you will need support, but you can do it.

Many years ago people with diabetes thought that they were doomed because complications came with the disease. That is not necessarily true! The complications are caused by *high blood sugar*, not from the disease. Therefore, if you keep your blood sugar well controlled, you can prevent or delay complications from occurring.

Bottom Line

You can prevent or delay complications by keeping blood sugar in your target range.

Know How Well You're Doing

You and your health care team can tell how well you are doing in your diabetes control by looking at three different parts of your diabetes care.

1. One of the ways that you and your doctor will know how well you are doing is by doing a blood test called HbA1c, or glycohemoglobin. That's a big word that basically measures how much sugar (glucose) is stuck on your hemoglobin (which is the part of a red blood cell). When you don't have diabetes, you have a HbA1c level of about 6 percent or less. When you have diabetes, however, the percentage can go much higher and that is one way your doctor determines how you have been doing over the past two months.

This blood test *should* run as close to normal as you can get it without having frequent or severe low blood sugar. Every little bit that you can drop the percentage will cut some of your risk of complications. Most people ask how they can get it down. The answer is to do whatever it takes to keep blood sugar levels within your target range.

The higher your HbA1c is, the more you are at risk for complications. So you should have this test done *every three months* at your doctor appointments to monitor how you are doing. If your HbA1c is extremely high, you may even need to have it checked between doctor appointments to make sure that it is coming down with changes in your treatment plan. There are now home test kits on the market that might help you test your HbA1c without going to a lab to have blood drawn. Ask your doctor if this is something that would work for you.

2. Glucose monitoring. Even if your HbA1c number is okay, you are not in good control of your diabetes if your blood sugar levels are bouncing between 40 and 400, or if they are consistently out of your goal range. The target range for blood sugars is to keep them normal, or basically 70–120mg/dl (your doctor will tell you what is best for you). If your numbers run consistently higher than that, don't accept that as being okay. Ask your doctor or diabetes educator what you can do to get them down.

3. Symptoms of diabetes or trips to the emergency room for diabetes problems also can show that you are not doing well. For example, if you have been having symptoms of high or low blood sugar, are getting up to go to the bathroom at night, are very thirsty, have a yeast infection, or are having frequent low blood sugar, your control is not what it should be.

Understanding Diabetes Complications

Diabetes can make other physical conditions worse, and other conditions can make diabetes worse. In the short term, for example, high blood sugar levels will cause an infection to take longer to clear up, and an infection will cause blood sugar levels to run high. It is, unfortunately, a vicious cycle.

Likewise, there are conditions that are more long-term. High blood pressure, for example, is a problem that can be caused by the effects of diabetes, but also when it occurs causes even more problems. Complications, when they happen, can be treated, but it is *much* better to keep them from happening in the first place!

It is neither smart nor healthy to dwell on the complications of diabetes. You will need to do for yourself what keeps you motivated and positive, rather than dwell on the negative things that could happen. However, it is smart to be aware that complications do exist, what they are, how to prevent them, and what to do if they occur. Some people might even try to scare you into doing what you need to do by using the threat of complications as an incentive to eat right or take care of yourself better. Has anyone ever told you, "If you eat that candy bar, your toes are going to fall off!" or "That cake is going to make you blind!" or some other such declaration? People who use scare tactics in this way usually mean well: they want you to take good care of yourself. But usually the threats are not helpful and don't motivate most people. It is true that having constant high blood sugar does cause complications of diabetes. It is also true that sweet foods cause blood sugar levels to rise. The problem is that when that candy bar is staring you in the face, it is hard not to eat the candy now, even though you are reminded that someday you might have to have your toes amputated. "Someday" seems awfully far away . . .

You might want to show people who use scare tactics how they can better help you do what you need to do for yourself. Many teens and adults alike take good care of themselves because they are "into" their health and don't want problems. But then there are also many who can't seem to stick to their program. We all need all the help we can get. Therefore, you could suggest some helpful ways this caring person can be more helpful, such as, "It is hard for me to have candy bars around and not eat them. I'd prefer it that you don't buy them, but if you do, keep them somewhere where they are not in my face, tempting me!"

We all (and teens are no exception) usually do what is personally important for us to do. If taking good care of yourself and your health is not important to you, you may need to ask yourself why that is the case and work to change that attitude. It is important to find what does motivate you if you are going to do this.

Since complications can occur with diabetes, your job is to cut your risks as much as possible, so you can prevent problems from happening. Complications can be prevented or delayed. It actually can be inspiring when you realize that a lot of what happens is up to you.

Diabetes complications can directly and negatively affect certain organs. Before you read on, remember that these do NOT need to happen to you. They don't happen suddenly, or without reason. *They are caused over time by long periods of high blood sugar.* They do not develop quickly, and that means they are not fixed quickly. Most teens with diabetes do not have any complications. But the beginning of complications can start with diabetes, and if your blood sugar control is poor, the damage can be happening to you without you being aware of it. Here are some of the complications that you may hear about.

HEART AND BLOOD VESSEL DISEASE

High blood pressure (hypertension) is a problem that is a danger to anyone, but is especially troublesome for someone with diabetes. Although the teen years are not usually a period when complications from diabetes occur, high blood pressure *can* show up during teenage years and should be treated. High blood pressure also is strongly associated with other complications of diabetes. For example, people who have heart disease, a high blood level of fats in their family, are obese, smoke, and have diabetes are all at risk for developing high blood pressure. Besides, people who have type 2 diabetes are already at risk because they are usually overweight, and therefore their risk of developing high blood pressure multiplies.

High blood pressure can cause damage to blood vessels. Also, it sets you up for damage to your heart, blood vessels, and kidneys. The longer you have high blood pressure, and the longer it is not treated, the better chance you might have of having a heart attack or stroke. Therefore, it is especially important to treat high blood pressure in the teen years, and to take steps to prevent high blood pressure from happening.

When you have your blood pressure taken, you will be told two different numbers. The top (or systolic) number is the higher one. This number is the amount of pressure your heart beat creates against the walls of your blood vessels. The second (or diastolic) number is lower than the first and is the amount of pressure against your blood vessels between heartbeats, when they are resting. The target range for blood pressure is to keep it below 120/80.

Although both numbers are important, the lower one is the one that is important to watch. If your resting pressure is always too high (for example, above 130/84), your blood vessels and heart can be damaged. The blood vessels become hard, clogged, or could leak, which causes strokes, heart attacks, and circulation problems in your feet.

When diabetes is not well controlled, and blood pressure is high, the blood vessels become damaged. Usually a blood vessel is elastic, like a rubber band, but over time, if it becomes clogged, it will lose its elasticity. Then, when blood pressure is high, the vessel can give out, or clog. It's similar to what would happen when enormous water pressure is present in an old hose: the hose might spring a leak and become damaged. If the leak happens in your brain, you could have a stroke. If it happens in your heart, or a vessel clogs, you could have a heart attack. Heart and blood vessel disease is the number one killer of people with diabetes.

However, the numbers shouldn't be completely based on what your blood pressure is in the doctor's office. Many people have "white coat syndrome," where blood pressure goes up when they get anxious, such as in a doctor's office. When your blood pressure is taken when you are more relaxed, it might be normal.

PREVENTING HIGH BLOOD PRESSURE AND HEART DISEASE

1. If your blood pressure is high, one of the first things you should do is cut the amount of sodium (salt) in your diet. (See Chapter 2, Pass on the Salt). Actually, it is the sodium that is the problem, but most of the sodium we eat comes from salt. Because salt helps the body retain fluid, when you eat foods high in salt, the volume of blood and other fluids increases. This causes blood pressure to go up. Remember the old hose attached to a spigot that has the water turned on full force? If the hose is old or damaged, the water pressure might cause a leak and actually damage the hose, like too much air in a balloon. Blood vessels are like the hose in that they can be damaged when blood pressure remains high for long periods of time. (See Heart and Blood Vessel Disease, page 99) When blood vessels are damaged, they become less elastic and begin to get fatty deposits on the inside. This can be the beginning of diabetes complications. If you are carefully cutting salt and your blood pressure still stays high (with the bottom number being greater than 84 mm), it might be time to start medication.

2. Keep your total cholesterol low! One of the types of fats in the blood is called *cholesterol*. People who have a high level of cholesterol are more prone to developing heart disease. Over time, the fats clog arteries and prevent blood from getting where it needs to go. When diabetes is out of control, the level of fat in the blood is usually high. The total cholesterol number is made up of "good cholesterol" (HDL) and "bad cholesterol" (LDL). These numbers are measured in a blood test, and the "good" type is a level that is thought to be protective against heart disease, while the "bad" type puts you at risk for heart and blood vessel disease. For people with diabetes, it is recommended that the "good" (HDL) cholesterol be higher than 45 mg/dl, and the "bad" (LDL) cholesterol be less than 100 mg/dl.

Your doctor should order that your cholesterol level be checked at least once a year. If your blood cholesterol is high, your doctor may tell you to cut back on food containing a lot of cholesterol, to exercise, and to improve your blood sugar control. If you are already doing that, without success in lowering it, then your doctor may need to prescribe a pill to help lower it.

(See the section on, "Understanding Fats," page 45).

Some foods high in cholesterol

Butter or lard
Egg yolks
Red meat, bacon, any marbled fat
The skin on chicken or turkey
Cheese
Whole milk
Lobster or shellfish
Lunch meats or hot dogs
Liver
Chocolate

---

3. Know your triglycerides! This is another form of fat, which is made in the liver from the food that you eat. As with cholesterol, when diabetes is out of control, your triglyceride level might be high. When you have a high triglyceride level, you are more prone for blood vessel disease such as strokes, ministrokes, and heart problems.

A triglyceride level of 400 mg/dl or higher puts you at risk for large blood vessel and heart disease. A level below 200 mg/dl will put you at low risk. If your levels are high, you can help by:

➤ Improving your diabetes control
➤ Avoiding simple sugars and rich desserts
➤ Cutting the saturated fats you eat (see Understanding Fats, Chapter 2)
➤ Eating more high-fiber foods (see Increase Your Fiber, Chapter 2)

➤ Eating fish fat! Fish such as salmon, tuna, sardines, or swordfish steaks have an oil that has been shown to lower triglyceride levels.

➤ Lose weight, if you are overweight.

4. Keep a healthy weight. Being overweight can lead to high blood pressure. When you are overweight, your heart has to work too hard to pump the blood around your body. This puts a stress on both your heart and blood vessels.

5. Exercise! When you exercise, you give your heart muscle a workout. Like any other muscle in your body, if you work out regularly, you will build up your heart and make it strong with good circulation. Exercise helps you from developing high blood pressure by improving your circulation and helping to control your weight.

6. Don't smoke or chew! Nicotine, which is the addictive substance in tobacco products, constricts blood vessels and leads to high blood pressure. When you have diabetes, or are overweight AND smoke, your risk for heart disease and high blood pressure sharply rises.

7. Take medication if you need it! If you need to take a medication to control your blood pressure, it is well worth it. Most of the medications used to treat high blood pressure in teens with diabetes have very few side effects. If your blood pressure runs consistently higher than normal, your doctor will recommend that you take a blood-pressure-lowering medication.

Bottom Line

High blood pressure and high blood sugar are at the root of diabetes complications.

Tyrone's Story

As Sally talked about high blood pressure, Tyrone was thinking that as far back as he could remember, his family

*had talked about blood pressure. Of course, that was
probably because everyone in the family had high blood
pressure, especially the men. Tyrone had never known his
grandfather, who had died a long time ago, but the family
always talked about him. He also had diabetes, and had a
heart attack at the age of 45 and died. Of course that was
before much was known about how to treat diabetes and
prevent heart disease. Tyrone looked at his dad, who was
also overweight and liked to cook, and who didn't
exercise. He thought, "Maybe this whole thing will be good
for Dad's high blood pressure. I'm gonna get him eating
right and working out with me!"*

• **Eye Disease or Retinopathy**—When blood vessels in the
back of the eye leak and bleed, it can threaten one's vision, and
blindness can occur. The eye disease that comes with diabetes
occurs in stages. The earliest stage is not vision-threatening at
all, but an eye doctor can see the signs when he looks at the
blood vessels in the back of your eyes. Some stages of this disease
require a laser zap to keep vision from getting any worse.

Preventing it: You can prevent diabetic eye disease by controlling your blood sugar and seeing an eye doctor every year.
When you are at the eye doctor, your eyes should be dilated
with drops so that he can examine them well. If he notices the
beginning of the eye disease, blindness can usually be prevented
by tightening up diabetes control, and by laser treatments to the
eyes. In fact, this complication does not happen as much anymore because people know more about how to care for their
diabetes and to prevent blindness.

• **Nerve Disease or Neuropathy**—When high levels of
sugar affect the nerves for long periods of time, the nerves might
begin to not work well. Usually the nerves in the feet, hands,
and sexual organs are most noticeably affected, but the major
nerves to your stomach and heart can also be damaged. If you
have any feelings of "pins and needles," numbness, tingling, restless legs, or pain in your body, tell your doctor right away.

One of the big problems of having numb feet and legs is that you can injure your foot, step on something, burn yourself, or have a wound that you don't know about until it gets infected. (See Foot problems page 106). It is bad news to have a foot infection because if blood sugar levels are not in good control, the infection can be hard to get rid of. Some people who have had diabetes for a long time have both nerve and circulation problems in their feet. They may get ulcers and infections easily. In extreme cases amputation may be necessary. It is important to do all you can to keep this from happening.

Preventing it: You can prevent nerve damage by controlling blood glucose. When damage does occur, improving blood sugar control will help. If pain occur in your legs or feet, there are also medications that your doctor may give you to help. As a teen, you most likely will not experience significant nerve damage, but it is smart to stay in good control so that you can stay that way.

Impotence—This is the inability of a man to have or sustain an erection. This problem is related to the damage that can occur both in nerves and blood vessels. When the nerves and blood vessels to the sexual organs are damaged due to complications of diabetes, it can be difficult for a man to perform sexually.

Preventing it: As is true for all of the other diabetes complications, in order to avoid problems the best thing you can do to prevent impotence is to keep blood sugar levels, as well as your blood pressure, as normal as possible.

• **Kidney Disease (Nephropathy)**—The kidney's job is to filter blood and rid your body of things it does not want by excreting them out into the urine. You have two kidneys that do this work. Having either high blood sugar or high blood pressure or both together can damage the blood vessels over time. The tiniest vessels in the kidneys are called *tubules.* When they are damaged, they leak and don't work well. One test that your doctor should do for you every year is to ask you for a sample of your urine to see if you have any kidney damage. This test looks for very small amounts of protein in your urine, called microalbumin. If you have an abnormally high amount of microalbumin in your urine, you could have the beginning of kidney disease.

Preventing it: Keeping your blood glucose level well controlled, and keeping your blood pressure well controlled, can prevent or delay kidney disease. You may need to take a medication to control blood pressure that will also help save further damage to your kidneys. When kidneys become extremely damaged, some people need kidney transplants in order to survive.

• **Foot Problems**—A healthy teenager, even one with diabetes, does not usually have serious foot problems. But it is smart to know that foot problems can occur and what to do about them. Learn how to take good care of your feet so that problems will not happen to you!

When diabetes complications do occur, the nerves and circulation to the feet are affected. You develop poor sensation, a lack of feeling, and foot deformities. This complication usually does not happen in the teen years, but can occur after years of poor diabetes control. Sometimes open ulcers develop and are hard to heal. Wounds or injuries can get infected. Some older people with diabetes have to have amputations. So, even though it might not be a big issue for you right now as a teenager, it is important to get into the habit of checking your feet for problems so you can prevent difficulties if they should crop up.

Preventing it: Inspect your feet every day. Check for red marks, blisters, cuts, athlete's foot, cracks, and dry skin. If you see a problem, take action immediately! Treat athlete's foot with a foot product from your pharmacy. Clean cuts and cracks, and cover them with antibiotic ointment adhesive. Do all you can to prevent blisters. Tip: A mirror can help you see the bottom of your feet.

➤ Wash your feet every day. Dry them carefully and check between your toes for cracks.

➤ Use a foot cream or lubricating oil, especially on dry skin, but don't put it between your toes.

➤ Cut toenails straight across to prevent ingrown toenails.

➤ *Never* cut corns or calluses! Smooth down a callus with an emery board instead. *Do not* perform "bathroom surgery"!

➤ See your doctor for help in removing warts. Don't use over-the-counter wart removal products because they can cause tissue injury that might become infected.

➤ Go barefoot as little as possible! Even indoors you can stub a toe or step on something sharp.

➤ Always check the insides of your shoes and boots before putting your foot inside. You might prevent a foot injury from something inside your shoe, anything sharp or worn that might cause blisters, or a tack through the sole.

➤ Don't smoke. Smoking contributes to poor blood circulation because the nicotine constricts blood vessels.

➤ Wear comfortable shoes, break new shoes in slowly so that you don't get blisters, and alternate your shoes.

➤ Pay attention to red marks, blisters, scratches, or scrapes on your legs and feet. Keep them clean, and if they become red or painful, you see pus, or they won't heal, tell your doctor right away.

➤ Avoid extreme temperatures! Learn to test bathwater before sticking your foot in so that you don't accidentally get scalded. Don't walk on hot surfaces such as sand at the beach or cement in your bare feet.

➤ See your doctor or a foot doctor (podiatrist) for ingrown toenails or other foot problems.

Maria's Story

Maria glanced down at her sandals with her bright, frosted blue toenails. She liked different colored nail polish and owned piles of glittery polish in bright and weird colors. Rita teased her mercilessly about the nail stuff she bought, yet asked Maria to do her nails, especially when she wanted nails to match an outfit. Maria didn't mind because Rita was generous with her own stuff. Maria listened to Sally, and thought about how scary it would be not to be able to feel her feet. Maria remembered watching her Aunt Rosa, who couldn't feel her feet or legs from the knees down, always put her hand inside her shoes before

*putting them on, just to make sure there was nothing in
them that could damage her feet. "Boy, I don't want that
to happen to me!" she thought. Maria liked to go barefoot,
but then remembered how she had cut up her feet walking
on gravel. Once she stepped on a beer bottle top in the
grass and sliced her toe, and another time she'd stepped
on a piece of glass. She thought that maybe she'd at least
wear sandals from now on.*

• **Tooth and Gum Problems**—Just as diabetes affects all the
rest of your body organs and tissues, high blood sugar levels can
also affect teeth and gums. Gum disease is called *periodontal
disease* and when you have diabetes, you are prone to developing it. A gum infection, like any infection in the body, can
cause blood sugar levels to run high. And serious gum disease
can lead to tooth loss.

Preventing it: When you have diabetes, it is especially important to see your dentist regularly, and brush and floss your
teeth often to help avoid problems. If your gums bleed frequently
when you brush or floss, talk to your dentist.

• **Depression: An Emotional Complication**—Do you
think sleep is the best part of your day and night? Do you have
trouble pulling yourself out of bed? Do you feel like life is not
worth the hassle and that your friends and family don't understand you at all? Do you want to volunteer to be roadkill? How
about pond scum?

Everyone has the blues once in a while, but if you are truly
having thoughts like this, or bouts of the blues more than once
in a while, then you could be suffering from depression. Having
no energy, wanting to be alone, sleeping a lot, crying, getting
angry, or not finding any joy in your life are all possible signs.
Sometimes when teens are depressed they turn to drugs or alcohol. And sometimes drugs and alcohol *cause* depression!

Diabetes is one of the few diseases that requires a lot of effort
on the part of the person who has it in order to manage it.
Diabetes is not a disease where you can take a pill and forget
about it. And that is the problem—there is all the stuff you have

to do or not do. So sometimes life with diabetes can feel overwhelming. Being a teen is a tough job in the world today, and being a teen with diabetes can be even tougher.

Depression does not necessarily go hand in hand with diabetes, but if you have a tendency toward being depressed, sometimes diabetes can push you over the edge into depression. Depression is more common in teens with diabetes than in others. It also tends to run in families, so if other family members have depression, you may be more at risk. Therefore, it is really important that you be able to recognize if you are depressed and know what to do about it.

Ignoring the fact that you are depressed does not help. Taking control of your diabetes can help you be in control of the rest of your life, and that can help to fight your depression. One path many teens take in an effort to ignore depression is to turn to alcohol, tobacco, or drugs as stressbusters. And although you may temporarily feel better from these substances, the good feelings don't last. You can end up feeling even worse. (See Chapter 5, Avoiding Substance Abuse)

When you are depressed, it becomes difficult, if not impossible, to take care of your diabetes. Diabetes slips from being a priority for you. Usually if life is going well, diabetes cares goes well, too. When life isn't going well, diabetes care doesn't, either. Let's say your parents just grounded you, you flunked a class in school, and your girl/boyfriend just broke up with you. You may not have the mental energy to stay on top of your diabetes care and do what it takes to take good care of yourself. On the other hand, when you ace a final, hit a home run, or are generally on top of your game, it seems easier to fit good diabetes care into life.

If you find that you are experiencing signs of depression, it is important to talk to a family member, clergy, medical team member, guidance counselor, or other adult. It is important to get help when you need it. Sometimes talking to an unbiased, objective person who can be there to support you in your struggles is all that it takes to get over the hump and back into a happy life. Otherwise, it may take a combination of antidepressant drugs, together with therapy, to help. A number of excellent medications on the market today can help, and together with counseling, they work very well. By taking care of your mental state, you are also taking care of your diabetes.

Everyone can be down or a little blue once in a while. It is important for you to know that these feelings are common and happen to everyone at times. It becomes more of a concern, however, if you are experiencing sadness or anger more often, or if the feelings are so strong that they get in the way of the rest of your life. Having diabetes is not a picnic: it can be frustrating, difficult, and at times frightening. But there is every reason for you to hope that things will go well with you as long as you do your part in managing it.

If you find that negative emotions are getting in your way, don't hesitate to talk to someone. It can be hard to take the first step: As one teen put it, "I'm too depressed to do anything about my depression!" But acknowledging that you have a problem is key, and do not wait for someone to talk to you about it. Don't wait for someone to ask. *You* take the initiative!

A GUIDE TO SIGNS OF DEPRESSION

If you have any of these problems, talk to your parents or some-one on your medical team to see if you should be evaluated further.

➤ *Not doing well in school.* Failing grades or a drop in grades when you have usually done okay in school is a red flag. Yes, you know when you're slacking, and there may be other reasons for poor grades. Maybe you have too much on your plate to be able to work at your grades. But if you have usually done well and you don't seem to have the emotional energy to do what it takes, and are distracted or sleepy, you may also be depressed.

➤ *Unable to focus.* Do you notice that when you sit down to concentrate, you can't seem to collect your thoughts? You are distracted, sleepy, or agitated, and your mind wanders. When you can't focus, you may find that when you sit down to study or read, you don't get anything done or can't remember what you did.

➤ *Tardy or absent from school.* You don't know why, but you can never seem to get up in the morning. You don't want to go to school and either intentionally or unintentionally find yourself late to class, and always having to cover absences. You've missed about as much school as the school will allow and you don't care. Your priorities are not in your future.

➤ *No interest in friends or activities that you used to enjoy.* You used to be in clubs, play sports, or do things with your friends. Now you don't feel like doing those things anymore. You avoid your friends, and the things you used to like to do don't give you any pleasure. You've dropped away from people who support you.

➤ *Sleeping too much or unable to sleep at night.* You have insomnia and when you do sleep, it only arrives after a struggle. When you do get to sleep you wake up a lot and then you are tired all day. Or the opposite can be true, where all that you want to do is sleep! You can't get out of bed in the morning, and when you come home from school you take a long nap, until it is time to go to bed.

➤ *Eating too much or can't eat.* You feel bored, or that life and food are out of control. You lay around and snack a lot. Food becomes a comforter and you have gained weight. Other people, when sad or depressed, are unable to eat and then lose weight.

➤ *Having trouble getting along.* You find yourself annoyed, agitated, frustrated, or in conflict with your parents, teachers, siblings, or even friends. You feel as though you are always fighting or quarreling about something with people you used to get along with pretty well.

➤ *Crying a lot.* You don't know why you are sad, but you find yourself either crying or feeling like crying a lot. You may cry yourself to sleep at night, or burst into tears easily.

➤ *Angry a lot.* Sometimes things in life mount up and can make you angry. If you find that you are frequently losing your temper or feel like losing it over both big and little things; are getting into trouble with your parents, teachers, or other authority figures; or find yourself arguing and fighting, you may need help.

➤ *Feeling sad or hopeless.* When life feels like too big of a struggle, is not worth living, or you have no hope of feeling better anytime soon, you may be feeling what has been described as the "blues." Ask someone to help you.

➤ *Feeling like hurting yourself or someone else.* If you have thoughts of injuring or killing yourself or someone else, it is of utmost importance to find help right away. Even if you are "only" entertaining the thoughts but have no serious intention of doing it, this is a sign that you should talk to a counseling professional right away. Tell your doctor or some responsible adult about your thoughts. Do not wait for someone to ask.

Bottom Line

Get help if you need it!

An Associated Illness: Thyroid Disease

"What's the thyroid?" you ask. The thyroid gland is in your neck, around your "Adam's apple" or larynx. (See Figure 7).

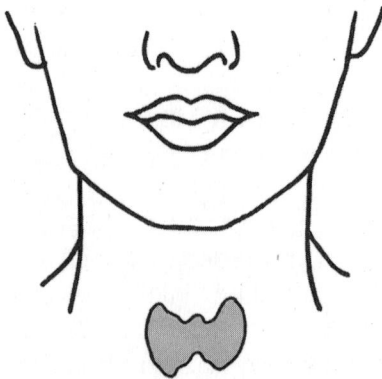

Figure 7: Thyroid gland.

It's job is to make thyroid hormone, which has the job of regulating how well your body burns food for fuel. Technically, thyroid disease is not a *complication* of diabetes, but it does commonly *occur* in people who have diabetes. People who have either type 1 or type 2 diabetes are more likely to develop a thyroid problem than others. When there is not enough thyroid hormone, it is called *hypo*thyroidism, and when there is too much, it is called *hyper*thyroid. Neither condition is healthy, but being *hypo*thyroid is more common in people with type 2 diabetes.

There is nothing that you can do to prevent thyroid disease from happening. If you have it, however, it is easily treatable. Your doctor should order a yearly screening test for thyroid function levels.

Here are signs of hypothyroidism.

➤ *Feeling cold.* Do you notice that you are uncomfortably cold when others are not? Do you need a sweater or extra blanket when others feel comfortable?

➤ *Tired.* You may feel tired all the time, sleep more often, and not be able to get up in the morning.

➤ *Weight gain.* Without any changes in your diet and exercise, you may find that you are gaining weight.

➤ *Constipation.*

➤ *Dry skin.*

➤ *Hair loss.* You may notice a lot of hair in your hairbrush or in the shower after you wash your hair.

➤ *Irregular periods.* If you are female, your menstrual periods may be irregular.

➤ *Goiter.* A goiter is an enlargement of the thyroid gland in the neck. Sometimes it can become tender or uncomfortable.

➤ *Poor growth.* Thyroid hormone is necessary in order to grow. Therefore, if your thyroid hormones are too low during your growth spurt, you may not grow to your full height.

TREATING HYPOTHYROIDISM

The treatment for hypothyroidism is to take a prescribed pill every day. There are no side effects from taking the pill because it is replacing a hormone that your body normally makes. When you take a pill to treat hypothyroidism, your blood levels should be checked regularly to make sure you are taking the dose that your body needs. The dose you need may change over time.

If you are hypothyroid and take the pill Synthroid or Levothyroid to treat it:

1. Take it every day, on an empty stomach. It's best to allow at least 30 minutes between taking your pill and eating.
2. If you skip a dose, you can take it late, or take two pills the next day to make up for it. (This is not the best thing to do—try to remember to take your dose when you're supposed to.)

Maria's and Tyrone's Story

"Geez," Maria thought, after hearing about all of the problems that could happen. Tyrone sat still, kind of numbed, and said, "Wow! I didn't know it could be that bad! There are a lot of people in my family that have 'sugar' and I never knew that their problems were all from diabetes." Then he thought about the sex complication. Man oh man. Some days all he could think about was girls, and he didn't want anything messing up sex! Talk about depressing. "After all," he thought "I'm just getting going." His thoughts wandered to his most recent girlfriend, Jonelle.

Sally spoke up. "Well, that is why you are here. It doesn't mean that it is going to happen to you, that you would have any complication. But it is smart to know what could happen if you don't take good care of yourself. You are here to learn so that you can deal with your diabetes, make smart choices, and avoid the complications. The more you know about what could happen, the better. You know what your risks are and you can recognize problems early on and treat them."

Tyrone smiled in relief and asked, "Do you mean if I do everything you say, that none of that stuff will happen?" (He was thinking that he would set the record for taking good care of himself!)

"Of course, there are no guarantees, Tyrone. But if you follow the guidelines most of the time, you will cut your chances of having problems. That is what diabetes care is all about. It is about trying to cut your risks as much as possible. No, you shouldn't let diabetes run your life, but yes, you should try to fit diabetes into your life in the smartest possible way."

5

Dating . . . and Other Stuff

When you have diabetes, sometimes the disease or the pressure of having it can get in the way. Things that you normally do, like partying or hanging out with your friends, can affect your diabetes control. The goal is to fit diabetes into your life, not to have your life revolve around diabetes. Even so, there are things that you will need to do differently because you have diabetes. Diabetes can impact your safety and health during activities that are common for you to do, such as drinking, driving, and traveling. Also, you will need to decide how much and when to tell friends, dates, and others about diabetes. There are all kinds of things to think about.

Sexuality

The word "sexuality" does not just mean "sex" or "doin' it" or "going all the way." Sexuality refers to your mental, physical, and emotional development. It also includes your awareness of the changes that are taking place in your body as you grow into an adult. Sexuality actually begins at birth, and is affected by all your feelings and attitudes about being male or female as you grow. If you are a guy, it may include how you you feel about the dark fuzz growing on your lip, or if you are a girl, how soon you need to wear a bra. It also may include your thoughts about those you are attracted to, as well as feelings of arousal.

Your body grows and develops quickly during the teenage years. If you didn't grow or develop there would be something wrong! The changes occur at different rates and different ages in everyone. You probably know people your age who grew much earlier or much later than you. Everyone is different, and within certain limits, it is all quite normal. There are specific hormones that begin and continue your sexual development. They are also partially responsible for your attitude about the opposite sex, which sometimes changes suddenly from active "dislike" and avoidance to active "like" and attraction.

The way you look and relate to others can help form your feelings about yourself and the way you think of yourself. Type 2 diabetes should not hold back your growth and development. In fact, teens with type 2 diabetes often are taller and heavier than other kids their age. Teens who are overweight often feel that others are not very nice to them because they are fat.

Almost all teens feel picked on and vulnerable sometimes for various reasons. You cannot tell from looking at someone whether he or she has diabetes, but diabetes can affect how you feel about yourself and your relationships because it adds one more way you may be a little different than everyone else. And let's face it, most people don't like to be different. When you have diabetes, it adds other concerns in addition to the normal issues of growing up. For example, maybe you have zits, or are too short, or too tall. Some teens may not like their hair or their build. Guys might feel too hairy or not hairy enough, or think they are too skinny or short. Girls are usually taller and heavier than the boys the same age are, and so they feel fat. Almost everyone has something about their appearance that bothers them.

As you develop into a man or woman, you learn to deal with a growing body and the effects of the hormones that make you grow. These hormones can cause you to develop acne, have mood swings, and, when you have diabetes, have insulin resistance. On top of this, there may also be pressures to be sexually active.

But did you ever notice that after you get to know someone, you don't really think a lot about what they look like anymore? Often you see looks first, but after that it is the whole person that you know. At first you might notice that he or she is overweight, but after you get to know the person you learn that he or she is fun, nice, smart, well-groomed, sharp and/or have a great sense of humor. Sometimes it is *self-confidence* that is attractive, and self-confidence can be sexy!

Sexuality, Self-Esteem, and Diabetes

Some of the concerns that teens with diabetes have relate to how their friends and dates will react to someone with diabetes. Most of the time it isn't a problem, but you may need to teach them a little about it. Some friends may need to be assured that they won't "catch" diabetes. If you take insulin, there also is the issue of taking injections or getting what you need when ordering food without making a big deal of your diabetes. Usually simple explanations work, but you may need to teach your friends what is going on in your life.

Since most teens with type 2 diabetes tend to be overweight, sometimes there can be problems with self-esteem because of extra weight. Society today puts a big premium on being thin. On the other hand, most people will respond to you because of who *you* are. Your attitude about yourself and your self-confidence affect how others respond to you. If you are positive, fun, and upbeat, other people usually will be as well. If you are negative and down on yourself, others might be down on you also. Part of your sexuality is how you present yourself to others. If you think you are a nice guy, others are likely to think so as well. If you act as if diabetes must be respected but is not an issue, others are likely to think the same. That is the image you need to put out there.

Bottom Line

Don't let diabetes change the way you feel about yourself.

Sexually Transmitted Disease (STD)

Teens who choose to be sexually active face two risks. First, if you are sexually active, you are at risk for getting common sexually transmitted diseases (STD). Second, these infections often have long-term, even lifelong effects. If you are sexually active, you should have, at a minimum, a yearly screening for STDs. People with diabetes are more at risk for infections of any sort, and may have a difficult time recovering from an infection when blood sugar levels are high. Infections in general, either viral or bacterial, can cause blood glucose levels to rise. But not every infection is caused by an STD. (See More Female Sexual Concerns.) However, if an STD is left untreated, there can be long-term problems from having it, even when it has been treated. Any infection, especially repeated and untreated ones, can lead to a serious condition called pelvic inflammatory disease (PID), which occurs in women. See your doctor right away if you are having any signs of an STD.

Signs of Infection

Open sore or discharge
Itching, burning, or irritation
Discomfort or pain in the genital area
Painful intercourse
Abdominal pain or tenderness (women)
Foul-smelling, yellow, white, or brown drainage
Swelling of sexual organs

Female Sexual Issues

It is important that you, a young woman with diabetes, have a knowledgeable woman to talk to when you have concerns or questions. It can be your mother, a favorite aunt, teacher, or someone on your health care team. When you have diabetes, almost every part of life is affected by it in some way, and that includes your sexual behavior. If you have poor diabetes control, your menstrual periods can be affected, or you may develop infections such as yeast. Women with diabetes also must be concerned about getting pregnant because high blood sugar levels affect the life and health of the baby. And women with diabetes are more prone to yeast infections and polycystic ovary syndrome, which we'll cover in a moment. First, here are the questions that women with diabetes frequently ask.

1. *Will diabetes affect my menstrual periods?* Answer: It can!
When you have diabetes, with reasonably controlled blood sugar levels, menstrual periods are likely to be completely normal. If diabetes is poorly controlled, periods might be irregular. If your menstrual cycles are always irregular, meaning that you could skip a month or two at a time, or have two periods in one month's time, your doctor may want to test your female hormones.

2. *Will my periods affect my diabetes?* Answer: Maybe
The jury is still out on this one. Some women report that they notice their blood sugar levels are higher than usual for a few days before and during the first few days of a period. Careful tracking of both blood glucose levels and menstrual cycles can help you to find a pattern. If you know that you have a pattern and you are on insulin, ask your doctor if you need an insulin dose adjustment for those specific days. Many women seem to eat differently prior to their menstrual periods, and it could be that extra snacking or the different foods alone are what causes blood sugar to be high. In any case, exercise is one treatment that can help improve high blood sugar, and can also be a stress-

buster! Think about trying some strenuous exercise during these times.

3. *Will I be able to have children?* Answer: Yes!! Most definitely.

Women with diabetes can get pregnant as easily as anyone else. However, it can be dangerous for you and your unborn child if your blood sugar is not in control for several months before and during pregnancy. It is extremely important that you plan your pregnancy so that you and your baby will be healthy.

When you decide that it is time for you to have a child, talk to your doctor so that together you can work to make blood sugar numbers as close to normal as possible for at least three months *before* you get pregnant. Then you will need to do whatever it takes to keep blood sugar normal during pregnancy.

Like women with gestational diabetes, a form of diabetes that happens during pregnancy, women with type 2 diabetes strictly follow a meal plan and might need to take insulin. Even if you currently treat your diabetes with a pill, you will need to take insulin during your pregnancy. You might go on an insulin pump or multiple daily injection program (four injections a day) to keep blood glucose levels normal for three to six months before getting pregnant.

Bottom Line

Plan your pregnancy so that you and your baby are healthy.

---

4. *What could happen to my baby if I don't take care of myself when I'm pregnant?* Answer: You may have complications during your pregnancy, and your baby may be sick or deformed.

Women with diabetes are more prone to complications of pregnancy, such as toxemia, where blood pressure goes up and you retain a lot of fluid. Complications can also include high blood pressure, premature delivery, and infection. If blood sugar runs high throughout pregnancy, the baby is also likely to have low blood sugar after birth. This is because the baby's pancreas overproduces insulin in response to its mother's high blood sugar.

Babies of mothers with diabetes also are often quite large at birth (over 9 pounds), even though they may be born on time or early. This is caused by mother's high blood sugar causes the baby to overproduce insulin, which causes weight gain. The baby is often full of extra fluids caused by faulty glucose regulation. Sometimes, even though they are big, they can have immature lungs and may have difficulty breathing at first.

The good news is that today, with good prenatal care, women with diabetes can have healthy pregnancies and healthy babies. It is not easy to do, but it is important to plan pregnancy and tighten up blood sugar control ahead of time. It will take discipline and motivation to keep blood sugar levels well controlled during pregnancy, but the outcome is a healthy mother and a healthy baby.

Pregnancy also can cause complications of diabetes in someone who has had poor control. The problem is that if you just get pregnant, don't know it, and haven't planned your pregnancy, having high blood sugar during the baby's early stages of development can cause birth defects and other serious problems.

5. *What if I'm sexually active and I don't want to be pregnant?* Best answer: Change your decision and don't be sexually active. Otherwise, use protection, meaning a condom and foam or gel.

Abstinence is the only completely safe sexual practice. Even the most reliable birth control method is not 100 percent safe in preventing pregnancy. Pregnancy is one of the biggest sexual issues concerning teens today. Teens who have babies before finishing high school are less likely to graduate and have the lifetime burden of being a single mother. Certainly, having a high school diploma can help to earn an income that is especially important when you have a baby to support. Many girls realize the difficulty that having to raise a child would be for them.

As a young woman today, you have a choice about your body. You can choose to be sexually active or not. Many teens are deciding that they aren't ready to have sex. They make this choice for a variety of reasons.

When you have the additional burden of having a disease like diabetes, ask yourself the hard questions about whether you are really ready and mature enough to handle pregnancy, diabetes, *and* a baby. As Sharon, a mature, pretty 15-year-old with type 2 diabetes put it, "I just couldn't deal with a baby yet. Sometimes I can't even take care of myself! How would I take care of a baby? A baby would really complicate my life. That's why I'm not taking any chances."

6. *What about birth control?* Answer: Abstinence is the safest birth control method. Otherwise, use a condom (a "rubber") even if you use other birth control methods.

Obviously, the best way to prevent pregnancy and sexually transmitted disease (STD) is to abstain from sex. Abstinence is the only 100 percent safe way of preventing pregnancy. Condoms can protect you from getting a sexually transmitted disease and from getting pregnant, but they are not foolproof. A tear, a leak, or early removal can mean bad news. In spite of what goes on in the movies and on TV, many girls today are making the decision to save themselves for their husband someday. It often takes a lot of maturity to make that decision and stick to it.

Carrie, a 17-year-old high school senior, put it this way: "I know my boyfriend, Gary, would like to have sex, but I thought about it and decided that I really want to save myself for my husband someday. I love Gary, but I don't know yet whether he's the one I want to spend my life with. I think it's really nice to stay pure for the guy I decide to marry. At least that's the way I feel about it right now. I think that Gary respects that, too. If he didn't, I wouldn't think that he really cared about me. I mean 'me,' the inner me."

The decision whether or not to have sex should be your *own*. Pressure from a girlfriend or boyfriend should not influence your decision. Ask yourself if you are ready to handle sex, and have a child, if you should become pregnant. These issues can be great topics of conversation for church youth groups, YMCA, scouts, and other groups where a responsible adult can guide the discussion.

If you are sexually active, it is very smart to choose to be protected. There is no such thing as completely safe sex. And having unprotected sex is stupid! When you do not use the protection of a condom, you expose yourself to HIV (the virus that causes AIDS), sexually transmitted disease, and/or pregnancy. Sexually transmitted diseases are syphilis, gonorrhea, chlamydia, genital herpes, and human papilloma virus (HPV, or genital warts). These diseases can have long-term effects, especially if they are not treated early. They can cause sterility and a potentially serious illness called pelvic inflammatory disease in women, which is an infection of your sexual organs and your gut.

7. *Can I use a birth control pill if I have diabetes?* Answer: Yes, if you don't smoke.

Birth control pills, or "the Pill," are one effective way to prevent pregnancy. This is called oral contraception (OC) and contains the female sex hormones, estrogen and progesterone. These hormones cause the ovaries not to release an egg each month, and cause the lining of the uterus to prevent an egg from attaching. You cannot become pregnant without a fertilized egg, so there is no pregnancy.

If you don't miss taking your daily pill, it can be over 99 percent effective in preventing pregnancy. The types of pills that are used are low doses of hormones that do the job of preventing pregnancy, but prevent some of the side effects of larger doses. However, if you have high blood pressure, heart or liver disease, cancer, or a strong family history of strokes or blood clots, the Pill may not be a good choice for you. If you smoke, you are not a good candidate for the Pill. Women who have diabetes, smoke, and are on birth control pills are at high risk for blood clots or strokes. You will need to talk to your doctor about the best choice for you.

There are also some side effects from taking birth control pills. These usually fade over time, but you may notice: a small weight gain, headache, breast tenderness or enlargement, nausea, mood changes, fluid retention, or spotting. Sometimes they can also make blood glucose levels rise. Some women with diabetes need to take the Pill to regulate their menstrual cycles.

Other ways of taking female hormones to prevent pregnancy are:

➤ An injection, better known as "depo," works for three months at a time. (This is also known as Depo-Provera or medroxyprogesterone acetate suspension, USP). While this is a very effective way of preventing pregnancy, it can also cause heavy bleeding during the periods of some women.

➤ A slow release from a device implanted under the skin. (Norplant System, levonorgestrel implants). It is 99 percent effective in preventing pregnancy. Your doctor must implant it. A downside of this system is that it can cause weight gain.

Keep in mind that although taking the Pill and other forms of birth control such as these can be effective in preventing pregnancy, only a condom can prevent you from getting HIV or an STD. Therefore, it is important to use a condom even if you are on the Pill, Depo, or Norplant.

8. *What about other kinds of birth control?*

Again, remember that birth control methods can prevent pregnancy, but will not prevent you from getting HIV or STDs. A contraceptive foam or gel should always be used with a condom so that you have a little insurance in the case of a tear, a leak, or coming off early.

A family planning clinic can help you with information and guidance, and answer your questions about birth control or other sexual problems. Many clinics have no fees and are confidential. Your doctor or someone on your medical team should be able to help you find one in your area.

Bottom Line

Abstinence is the only 100 percent protection from pregnancy and sexually transmitted disease. Protect yourself!

Your options are:

- *Diaphragm*: a soft rubber cup that fits over the entrance of the uterus. It is 85–97 percent effective in preventing pregnancy and is most effective when used with a spermicidal jelly. The drawback to its use is that it must be inserted in advance, or lovemaking must be interrupted.
- *Sponge*: an absorbent sponge that acts as a barrier to sperm. It is 90 percent effective in preventing pregnancy. It also must be inserted in advance, or lovemaking must be interrupted. It can stay in place for six hours after having sex.
- *Depo-Provera* (sterile medroxyprogesterone acetate suspension, USP): an injection of a hormone that works for three months to prevent pregnancy. It is 99 percent effective in preventing pregnancy. The drawback is that it can cause irregular or heavy bleeding during a period.
- *Norplant* (levonorgestrel implants): a device implanted under the skin that gives a continuous release of hormones. It is 99 percent effective in preventing pregnancy. Drawbacks are that a doctor must implant it and a side effect might be weight gain.
- *"The Pill"*: There are a number of brands of female hormones that are taken on a daily basis. It is over 99 percent effective in preventing pregnancy when taken as directed. The drawback is that there can be side effects (See section 124, the Pill).

Other methods of birth control, such as rhythm, withdrawal, or temperature monitoring, are not recommended because they are not ideal for anyone. They only prevent pregnancy between 60 and 85 percent of the time when done properly. Another drawback is that these methods are either hard to control or inaccurate.

Bottom Line

Be safe and be careful if you choose to be sexually active.

Maria's Story

Maria listened intently, because she really wanted to get married and have kids someday, but certainly not soon. She felt somewhat relieved that diabetes wouldn't interfere with that. And all the stuff on birth control, well, that was a whole other issue. She hadn't really thought about it much, because she didn't have a boyfriend. Rita didn't have a boyfriend either, but a lot of their friends did and some were talking about sex. Maria knew two girls who had babies to take to school with them every day. She didn't know how they did it. She couldn't imagine taking care of a baby at this point. It was all that she could do to take care of herself! And what if the baby were sick or was deformed or something? Wow!

Maria wondered what she would do if she were faced with the choice of having sex. Her friends all thought it was something cool, if not exactly great yet. Mama and Papa had always drilled into her head that sex was to be saved for after marriage. Although she didn't really understand what was supposed to be wrong about sex before marriage, she noticed a lot of worry and stress in the kids who got pregnant.

Because they had been talking a lot lately about planning ahead, Maria thought about what she would do when the situation came up. It was probably a good idea to think about it and make a decision beforehand, and not when she and a guy were alone together. She also thought about how disappointed and upset her family would be if *she got pregnant and said to herself, "If I ever got pregnant, my parents would KILL me!"*

MORE FEMALE SEXUAL CONCERNS

Women with diabetes are prone to developing vaginal *yeast infections.* When blood sugar levels remain high, it is hard for the body to fight an infection. High blood sugar changes the acidity of the vagina and makes it a good place for yeast to grow. Many women can get a yeast infection after treatment with antibiotics. Also, wearing clothing that does not "breathe," such as nylon, spandex, lycra, or tight clothing, can cause the problem.

Signs of vaginal yeast infections are: itching, burning, discharge, or irritation in the genital area. The discharge may look like yellow or white cottage cheese.

The first time you have symptoms, you should see your doctor to make sure of the diagnosis. There are over-the-counter medications such as miconazole or nystatin that can be purchased, but be careful to avoid overtreatment with these products. If they don't work, your doctor can prescribe other medications. See your doctor if your treatment is not working. Some women who repeatedly treat for a yeast infection can develop a secondary infection called bacterial vaginosis, which requires a prescription drug to treat. Yeast also can be present with other infections, so it is important to see your doctor if you have symptoms.

You can prevent yeast infections by:

➤ wearing underwear with a cotton crotch (not cotton over nylon)
➤ wearing loose-fitting clothing with fabric that breathes
➤ avoiding bubble baths
➤ avoiding scented or deodorant sanitary napkins or tampons
➤ carefully controlling your blood sugar (especially during use of antibiotics)

Polycystic ovary syndrome (PCOS) is a disorder found in women where many cysts form on the ovaries. Okay, now you're asking, "What does this have to do with diabetes?" Well, all of the hormones in your body have some effects on other hormones. (This is how hormones work: one hormone will stimulate or shut off another one. They are interrelated!) The ovary is the female reproductive organ that makes and releases eggs and female hormones. Cysts on the ovaries can cause an imbalance of male and female hormones. When there is an abnormal production of two of the female hormones, the ovaries are prevented from releasing an egg each month, so menstrual periods are irregular. The hormone imbalance also results in an increased production of the male hormone testosterone. Therefore women who have this imbalance usually have signs of male sexual characteristics from too much testosterone.

Signs of PCOS are:

➤ Irregular periods
➤ Very light or very heavy bleeding during periods
➤ Infertility
➤ Excess hair on the face, chest, and abdomen
➤ Obesity
➤ Acne on the face, shoulders, and back

Women who have polycystic ovaries also are at risk for type 2 diabetes because the excessive hormones cause insulin not to work well (insulin resistance). Women who have this problem may be treated with birth control pills and/or metformin (Glucophage), which help to regulate the hormone imbalance and cause insulin to work better.

Women who are being treated for PCOS will usually notice that their periods become more regular, and their acne improves. The excess facial hair may grow lighter, but may not completely go away. Some women with this problem will have electrolysis done if remaining facial hair is a problem for them. If you have symptoms of PCOS, bring it to your doctor's attention so that blood work can determine if you have it or not.

Male Sexual Issues

Guys with diabetes are most often interested in knowing if diabetes will affect their sexual performance. As Lenny put it, "At age seventeen, sex was always on my mind!" The answer is that diabetes can affect your sexual performance, especially if blood glucose levels are uncontrolled.

When blood sugar runs high and you are dehydrated, tired, and not feeling well, your sex drive may be affected. This is not an ongoing problem, as is the complication of impotency, and does not differ from any other person who at times is tired, dehydrated, or sick. What is more of a concern, however, is impotency (which usually occurs after years of poor control). When the nerves and circulation to the genital area are affected, there is difficulty having or sustaining an erection. But psychological factors can also play a role in impotence, and alcohol or drug use, stress, depression, or medications can contribute to the problem.

Men with diabetes can take the following steps to prevent diabetes-related impotence:

- Improve your blood glucose control.
- Keep physically fit. An improved self-image can help improve sexual function.
- Seek counseling if you have signs of depression.
- Let your doctor know about any problems in this area. Most dysfunctions are treatable.

Impotency can be a big motivator for many men with diabetes to take care of themselves. As Lenny put it, "Some of those other complications seem way out there. But this one hits too close to home! I don't want diabetes messin' that up!" Lenny has gone on to be married, and now has three children. He has taken care of himself!

Tyrone's Story

Tyrone listened intently to the things Sally was saying. Wow! If he wasn't affected by any of the other problems that could happen, he sure was by this one! There was no way that he wanted this one! He was now more determined than ever to stay in good control of diabetes.

When It Comes to Friends and Dating . . .

Sometimes it is hard to know what and who to tell about your diabetes. You don't want to advertise that you have diabetes to the world, and yet what is the big secret? It takes some time and experience to sort out whom to tell about diabetes and whom not to. It doesn't mean that by not telling some folks you are hiding it or it is an embarrassment, but just that there is nothing to be gained by sharing the information.

Of course, your best friends ought to know about diabetes so that they can support you in your care. But when do you tell other people? And how do you let someone you go out with know about your diabetes? Everyone seems to handle it a little bit differently, and that's okay! Julie, for example, is right up front with everyone about her diabetes. She tells her dates what to expect before they even go out. Sometimes she even shows them her meter, and talks about healthy eating. ("If they have a problem with it, well, good-bye! Neither one of us is wasting our time.") On the other hand, Jeff is much more reserved about telling a friend about his diabetes. Sometimes he waits until he's offered candy or something, and then says, "Thanks, but I shouldn't eat that 'cause I have diabetes." That is his lead into his introducing the concept. Some people are very private and

---

Bottom Line

The best thing a guy can do to keep a healthy sex life healthy is to take good care of his diabetes.

others are much more open. There is no right and wrong way. The only bottom line is your safety.

This means that you will need to tell others enough so that you can do what you need to do to take care of yourself, and be safe. Part of what and how much you tell others will depend upon your management program. If you manage diabetes by watching your diet and exercise, it will not be necessary to tell everyone about your diabetes, unless you want to. It can be a good thing to share it with your friends and others, because it can help to keep you on your program if others know what your needs are. If you don't tell your friends that you shouldn't have sweet desserts, they may tempt you constantly with Twinkies, Jolly Ranchers, and regular soda. But if they know that you have diabetes, a friend might offer you a diet soda, sugar-free gum, or popcorn instead of cookies. If friends know that you are trying to lose weight for your health, they should support you in your efforts. When "friends" sabotage your efforts, you might wonder if they really are your friends. A true friend will want what is in your best interests.

As to who else you tell about your diabetes, you might think about it this way: There are people who need to know about your diabetes, others where it may be nice if they know about your diabetes, and others who do not need to know.

The folks in the "needs to know" category are those who are with you frequently and are responsible for your safety. This might include your family members, teachers, coaches, chaperones, or other adults in leadership positions. These people need to know that you have diabetes, recognize signs of high and low blood sugar, and be familiar with your treatment plan. They will need to know what to do in case of an emergency, where your supplies are, and who to call in an emergency. If you go on a field trip or band trip with your school, have an all-night lock-in with your church youth group, or sleep over at a friend's house, the adult present should be made aware of your needs. Again, if your treatment plan does not make you prone to low blood sugar, there may be very few people who need to know you have diabetes, because you will not require emergency treatment.

People who it's "nice" to tell might be those who could wonder what you're doing when they see you testing your blood sugar, or kids you spend time with who might be supportive of you. Your pastor, priest, or rabbi may not actually need to know about your diabetes for your health and well-being, but it might be nice to tell him or her so that you can receive some spiritual support and encouragement.

If you play the drums in the school band, your band director is in the "needs to know" category. The other drummers in your section wouldn't have to know about your diabetes. But if you have a chance of having a low blood sugar while you're wildly drumming away, or if the band only receives sips of regular soda at games, it would be nice if the others had an awareness of your diabetes. They could then be helpful in times of low blood sugar, and not tempt you with sweet drinks or food all the time. Otherwise, it should make very little difference to anybody.

People in the "don't need to know" category are those who don't have much regular contact with you and are not responsible in any way for your care. You probably have plenty of classmates in this category. There is no need to tell the cashier at the drugstore or people you meet at a party or football game, unless you want to. They would most likely never be in a position to help you, support you, or treat you in an emergency.

Telling a Friend About Your Diabetes

Here's an example that can help you get across what you need to say clearly.

• Explain what diabetes is and how it is treated. *"I have type 2 diabetes. My body cells can't use insulin to get sugar from the food that I eat. So then sugar stacks up in my blood and I can have a high blood sugar. If I eat right, and can lose weight, my blood sugars might improve. Right now I take a pill to control my diabetes. I have to test my blood sugar twice a day and exercise a lot. Otherwise, I'm completely fine and can do everything that you do. I need to keep my blood sugar in control so* that I stay well, and not develop physical complications in the future."

• Show how to test your blood sugar. *"I check my blood before breakfast and after dinner. First I wash my hands, then I do a little prick on my finger. My blood sugar should be around 70 to 120, but sometimes it can go higher . . ."*

• Tell them about your meal plan. *"It's especially important for me not to pig out and not to eat too many sweet desserts or candy. You can help me by encouraging me to eat healthy foods and follow my plan. Ask me if something (like chocolate milk or orange drink) is on my plan. Sometimes I can have stuff like desserts, and certain kinds of cookies, just not too much of it. But most of the time I should eat healthy. That means fruits, vegetables, and watching the fat in my diet."*

• Tell them what to do if you take insulin or have low blood sugar. *"Because I take insulin to treat my diabetes, sometimes if I exercise or don't eat enough, I can feel a little shaky, sweaty, and hungry. If that happens I might be having a low blood sugar. My body is telling me that it needs sugar. I know it can be confusing that most of the time I can't have sugar, then suddenly I need it, but that's the way it is. Sometimes things just aren't balanced."*

Tyrone's and Maria's Story

Tyrone really didn't see much need to tell anyone about his diabetes right now. He was always kind of a free thinker, and wasn't influenced too much by what other people said or did. But as he thought about it, he decided that since he hadn't known about diabetes, maybe the other kids didn't know anything about it, either. Suddenly he thought it was important for people to know. After all, this pamphlet in front of him said that there were an estimated 17 million Americans with diabetes. Then he thought about the paper that he was going to have to write and present next month. Maybe he'd do it on type 2 diabetes and teach his class about it. He thought that if the class knew that he had diabetes, they'd be really interested.

Maria was thinking about Rita and how much she loved her company. Rita was truly a best friend, and would help her tell everyone about diabetes in a way that was positive. She could count on her and knew that Rita would help her do what she needed to do. Maria hoped that she could be that kind of a friend for Rita someday if need be.

Telling Your Date About Your Diabetes

Teens don't "date" much anymore. They just "go out" in groups or as couples. Still, there are things to consider about telling your group of friends, or when you meet someone of the opposite sex. One question that often comes up is "when to tell" someone about your diabetes. Do you tell about it up front and risk "scaring them off" (as one teen said)? Or do you wait until you are well into a relationship and then spring it on them? Neither of these ways seems like a great solution. The best answer is to talk about it after you get to know a person a little, but before the friendship becomes a relationship. Hopefully you will be able to find a way that works best for you.

Safety remains the main issue here. Again, if you take insulin or are on a medication that can make you hypoglycemic, it is very important that the people around you know what to do if you have symptoms. But even if you manage your diabetes with diet and exercise, it is a healthy approach to tell your date that you have special needs. It would be no different if a smoker asked someone out who had asthma. It is only right that there be an open and honest discussion sometime early in the relationship if safety is a factor.

Besides, if you are spending a lot of time with someone, it is important that he or she know what is going on with you so that there are no surprises, and also so that he or she can support you. A boyfriend or girlfriend can be a huge help in your care because he or she is someone who genuinely cares about you. Of course, parents and siblings care about you also, but sometimes because of the well-known parent/teen struggles, you may do better with a friend who is trying to help keep you on track. It is a matter of whatever works! If your boyfriend reminds you to test your blood, asks what your numbers are, and can get you to go for a walk with him, that is GREAT!

You may not want to hear this, but it is not unusual for your greatest help to come from your parents in spite of the fact that you occasionally feel nagged. However annoying it is, the nagging is for a good reason, and if you want to get the nagger off your back, you may need to start showing them that you are doing what you need to do to take care of yourself. You might even ask your mom or dad to check on your blood sugar numbers every day, or not to leave the candy in a place where you are tempted to eat it every time you pass by.

Maria's and Tyrone's Story

Sally told them a story about one girl's first struggles with telling her boyfriend. (She told them that names were changed to protect "the innocent.")

Shauna, a 15-year-old African-American girl with type 2 diabetes, was invited to the prom by Lemont. Since she hadn't had diabetes very long, she didn't have experience in knowing what she could and couldn't safely do. Shauna managed her diabetes with diet, exercise, and insulin.

She was really excited because this was the first time she had ever been asked out, let alone been able to go somewhere as exciting as a prom! And Lemont was pretty cool. In fact, he was awesome. Shauna's older sister, Val, was going to loan her a great dress, and help her do her nails and hair. The only thing that worried Shauna was that Lemont wanted to go out to dinner with others before the prom and said he'd pick her up about four o'clock. Shauna hadn't thought about it at the time because she was so excited to be asked, but then remembered that she had to take her insulin before dinner. She wondered how she would test her blood sugar, take her insulin, eat, and manage it all, since Lemont didn't know about her diabetes.

And since she didn't know him that well, she didn't want to tell him about it. She fretted and fussed about it all until Val said, "What's the BIG DEAL? Why don't you just tell him you have diabetes? If he changes his mind, that's HIS loss. Why would you want to go with someone like that, anyhow?"

Shauna had been tempted not to tell him at all about her diabetes, but then thought that it wouldn't be too cool if she had a low blood sugar while dancing. That could really ruin things. She could go into the restroom and test her blood without him knowing, but she would have to carry her stuff and hope he didn't wonder what it was. She guessed that it would be best if she would just talk it.

Shauna saw Lemont the next morning and asked if she could talk to him for a minute. They walked over to the corner of the hall and as she put out her hand to steady herself against the lockers, Lemont noticed her medical ID bracelet and said, "I've seen you wear that before. What's it for?" Whew! "Great lead-in," Shauna thought. "Well," she stated, "that's what I wanted to talk to you about. I thought you should know that I have diabetes, and that when we go out, I may have to test my blood sugar and take insulin." She blurted it out.

Lemont just looked blank. "Sooooo . . . ?"

"Well, I thought you should know. Plus, if my blood sugar drops, I might need to drink sugar or something. I'll tell you all about it later, if you want to know."

"Okay." Lemont looked a little confused, as though he was missing something. Shauna was relieved. He hadn't said "forget it," and seemed willing to work with her. It hadn't been nearly as big a deal as she had imagined.

Sally continued, "The point is that most people won't care that you have diabetes, and if you take the time to explain what you need to do, people won't think twice about it. But it's important to tell the people you spend *time with about diabetes so they can support you and care for you in case there's an emergency."*

When It Comes to Partying . . .

Celebrating with friends is a part of life. Diabetes should not get in the way of doing the things you want to do. You will learn how to handle holiday parties, all-nighters, sleepovers, and the fun that comes with them. You will also need to learn how to take care of your diabetes along the way. Sometimes it isn't easy, and sometimes your blood sugar may not be perfect, but it is important to do the best you can to keep your blood sugar within your target range. A diabetes educator can help you if you aren't sure how to adjust your food, schedule, exercise, or medication.

Going to a party or celebration or just getting together with friends is a great way to celebrate and have fun. There is no reason that you shouldn't participate because you have diabetes. You can party even with your diabetes program of following a meal plan and controlling your weight. The key to being successful in doing what you need to do in controlling your eating is in being prepared.

Here are some tips that may help you stay in control.

• Find out ahead of time what is being served. You can then plan what you will eat for the day, including the food you want to eat at the party.

• Be assertive in asking the waiter or waitress about foods on the menu. Find out if they are fried or if the restaurant carries sugar-free syrup, for example. Ask what comes with the meal. You may not know what comes with the meal and may not want it all. Most restaurants will be happy to assist your special requests. Airlines also offer low-fat, low-cholesterol, vegetarian, and diabetes meals.

• Offer to bring a healthy food to a party or get-together. You can bring something that fits into your program, and this way you know there will be something there that you can eat.

• Make sure that there is sugar-free soda on hand, or bring your own.

Admittedly, it is often a pain to have to watch what you eat during a special occasion. Party foods are usually not low in calories! But with your new knowledge about healthy eating, you can try to make smart choices. For example, go for the baked chips with salsa instead of regular chips with sour cream. Eat the veggie pizza instead of pepperoni and sausage with double cheese. Eat raw veggies with a low-cal dressing. Have plain bread instead of croissants, and bagels instead of doughnuts, to avoid extra fat. Get the idea?

Sometimes you may choose to eat things over and above what is on your usual plan. Once in a while, it is okay to do so. However, diabetes can sometimes give you a nasty reminder that you can't always do what you want to do when you want to do it. The key is not to eat so many calories that it will take a week of discipline to balance them out.

And with today's small, quick meters, it is pretty easy to test blood sugar on the run or at a party. When your blood sugar control is out of whack, you may not feel well, and that surely isn't welcome at any celebration.

Bottom Line

Don't let party time put a crimp in your future!

Maria's and Tyrone's Story

Both Tyrone and Maria were getting restless. They had been sitting listening to Sally for an hour, and Tyrone's leg was aching.

Suddenly Tyrone's dad spoke up, asking Maria, "Okay, young lady. All of this stuff about parties and goodies. How are you going to be able to do it? I'd like to hear from you, so that Tyrone can see how someone else will deal with it." Maria looked at Mama, then Rita, but both were silent. Maria then looked at Tyrone, and thought that Tyrone probably had a better handle on it than she did.

"Well, I'm not really sure yet until the situation comes up . . ."

"But aren't we supposed to anticipate? Plan ahead?"

Maria's dad jumped in at that point, saying, "Maria, you and Tyrone are going to have to make decisions about how you will handle things far ahead of time so that you'll be ready and not get caught off guard when you are tempted with something. If you decide now how you will handle things ahead of time, you'll already have worked through the decision and how to handle it. It will be easier to stick to your guns when something comes up."

Tyrone spoke up quietly just then. "Well, when it comes to booze, I think I'll just avoid putting myself in those situations."

Dad then said, "Son, that might work for some situations, but you can't just avoid food and you shouldn't avoid celebrations. You can't put yourself in a bubble for the rest of your life! Besides that, why punish yourself if you enjoy celebrating with your friends? There are enough punishments in life! Just learn to take care of yourself while you go to the party, and you will still have a good time."

Maria was sitting there in amazement after Tyrone's comment. "Tyrone has some kind of will power," she thought. Not go to a party to protect your blood sugar? No way! She said aloud, "I'll NEVER not go to a party! But, of course, I know I'll probably eat everything in sight!"

Rita said firmly, "No! You can't! We'll do what we plan to do. Look, I'm not going to eat stuff, either. Or I'm going to drink sugar-free soda and be really careful. If I can do it and I don't have diabetes, you can do it for yourself and your diabetes."

Sometimes Rita could be an awesome friend. After all, Rita didn't even have diabetes, yet she was acting like she *did. Still, Maria thought, "But she doesn't have to stick her finger and take shots! And she doesn't have to worry about getting sick. And she knows that if she doesn't stick to it, nothing bad will happen." However, that didn't take away from how nice it was of Rita to help her by sharing all the stuff she was going through.*

Overnighters

There are often opportunities to stay up all night, especially for teens. You may go to the prom (and after-prom activities), all-night bowling, a casual slumber party where no one sleeps, or a youth group "lock-in," or pull an all-nighter for exams. Somehow, all-night activities are far more attractive to teens than to adults! Part of the reason for this is actually grounded in our biorhythms, as it has been shown that when left to their natural body clock teens will stay up at night until the wee hours and sleep during the day.

When you have diabetes, especially if you take insulin to treat your diabetes, there are special things to think about when you stay up at night. If you take pills, maintaining a regular meal schedule is also important. One thing to remember is that since your body is up and active and not sleeping, you are spending more energy than you do when you sleep. That means it is very important to test your blood sugar and adjust food accordingly. If you find that your blood sugar is low while you are dancing or playing, you may need an extra snack. On the other hand, blood sugar might run high because you are awake and nibbling on pretzels or snacks.

The other thing to think about is what happens the next day when you crash until the afternoon. It is not smart to miss a dose of insulin, and it is also dangerous to take insulin and not wake up for meals and snacks. You will need to talk to a diabetes educator about the best way to handle this. It may be that you take part of your insulin, set the alarm, and get up and test your blood sugar. That's not the nicest thing to have to do, but it is the safest way of pulling an all-nighter without putting yourself in danger of having a low blood sugar. If you take pills, you will need to check with your doctor to find out what to do if you miss a dose or aren't eating a meal. What to do will depend on the specific pill you are taking. Don't forget to tell your friends a little bit about your diabetes and what they should look for in hypoglycemia, since they will be with you all night.

Chad's Story

Chad, a husky 16-year-old with type 2 diabetes, could sing, dance, and act. He was also a comedian. After starring in his class musical, Chad went to the cast party. As he took two types of insulin, before his dinner shot that night, he had lowered his dose by 10 percent, thinking that he would be active in the play and didn't have that much time for dinner. He had grabbed a half a sandwich going out the door, since he really didn't want to have a low blood sugar in the middle of the play. But he hadn't thought about the all-night activities afterward.

Chad performed well, and the show was great. Then they all went out to eat, dance, and party afterward, and suddenly Chad didn't feel so well. He felt very tired, but thought it was because it was late on a Friday night and he hadn't slept much all week. He hadn't brought his meter to test his blood sugar, and hadn't even thought about it. He walked over to some chairs near the food tables and sat down, putting his head in his hands. The next thing he knew, he was looking up from the floor and everyone was standing around him. The director, Mr. Eisen, was standing over him with an empty glass and Chad suddenly realized that his face was all wet and sticky from sugar. Mr. Eisen said he must have had a low blood sugar because he had fallen asleep and would not wake up. Chad had told Mr. Eisen about his diabetes at the beginning of play practice, so he knew what to do. But as there was no glucagon there, it was fortunate that he could get Chad to swallow some soda. After about 10 minutes

Chad was okay, but he vowed never to ignore his diabetes like that again. His friends told him later that at first they thought he was joking around the way he often did, but they became scared when they understood that there really was a problem. Chad was embarrassed, but felt lucky that his friends were kind and supportive. Since he wanted to consider a career in theater, he thought he should talk to a diabetes educator or his doctor to see what he did wrong, or how he should manage the next time. Later, his educator taught him that he should have cut back on his dinner insulin dose and tested his blood during and after the play, and then later at the party. Also, he learned that he should not have skipped his evening snack, but could have eaten food at the party.

Safe Driving

Being old enough to drive is almost like a rite of passage. It is the time of life when all at once you become independent and take on adult responsibility. When you drive, you have not only your own life but also everyone else's life in your hands.

When you have diabetes, there are some extra considerations that you will need to think about, especially if you take insulin. If you are not taking medication and have diabetes, the issues of driving are the same as for any other teen. You must be a responsible driver, and you must obey the law. With or without diabetes, it is obviously extremely important not to drink or use other substances and drive. Driving under the influence of alcohol does nothing for you, your driving record, or your future.

If you have diabetes and are taking medication, driving has some added hazards for you and everyone else on the road unless you are responsible about taking care of yourself. You may be particularly likely to have a low blood sugar if you take insulin or are on some of the oral agents (pills) to treat diabetes. Being low, or hypoglycemic, slows your reflexes in ways similar to drinking alcohol. When your blood sugar is low, you cannot make good judgments, nor can you drive safely.

Bottom Line *for everyone*

Don't drink and drive! Always wear your seat belt!

For teens with diabetes who take insulin or medication:

• Wear your medical ID. (See the section on "Wearing Medical ID," page 171.)

• Always test your blood sugar before getting behind the wheel.

• If you are on pills or insulin, make sure that you always have some snacks stashed away in your car in case of low blood sugar. Keep juice, crackers, and glucose tablets on hand. (Try not to eat your snacks if you are "just hungry" or bored while driving. If you eat them when you don't need them, you may not have them when you need them!)

• If you think you might be low, pull over and test your blood if possible. Have something to eat or drink.

• For long trips, stop and test your blood sugar at least every two hours if you take insulin, and take more supplies than you think you will need.

• Be careful storing insulin, strips, and meters in a very cold or hot car. Extreme temperatures can affect them. Insulin will lose its potency if it becomes frozen or hot. Meters may not work properly in extreme temperatures; check your individual meter's directions.

Maria's Story

Maria wasn't quite old enough to drive yet, but she had already thought about what it would be like. "I can't wait!" she thought. "It will be so cool!" She didn't think that having diabetes would be a problem for her. She planned to do everything she was supposed to do to take care of herself. Sally then told her a story.

"I know a girl who has type 2 diabetes, and takes the pill metformin and insulin. We'll call her Kate. She's 17

*and got her license last fall. I think it was in December
that Kate left work for the short trip home. She tested her
blood sugar before she left for home. It was a perfect 110
mg/dl and she hopped in the car. That was one of the
days we had a huge ice storm, and it caused a 14-car pile-
up on the freeway. She got stuck in traffic for over three
hours. Kate started feeling shaky and sweaty and ate the
two glucose tablets left in the glove compartment. She had
forgotten to restock her supplies. At first she had kept an
emergency box in the trunk, but since she had never
needed it, she had taken it out and put it in the garage so
she'd have more room in the car. She figured that she was
never that far away from home, a vending machine, or a
store. Now, however, she still felt low and started to be a
little fearful that her blood sugar would drop even more.
She searched her purse, the glove compartment, and under
the seat again. She found a Tootsie Roll pop that her
brother had left in the back seat and ate that. After ten
minutes she still felt low, and traffic wasn't moving at all.
There was nothing else in the car or her purse, so she
had to get out of the car and try to find food in the
surrounding cars. She approached the drivers in the cars
around her and told them her problem. She was lucky! The
guy two cars away found his kid's roll of Life Savers. Kate
learned her lesson. She was both relieved to have gotten
through the situation, and lucky. Now she keeps her car
well stocked with juice, glucose tabs, and crackers."*

*Maria thought that the story was amusing, but it did
have a point. She would hate to have to be bumming food
from others on the freeway. How embarrassing! She
thought about a blue nylon zippered bag that she had at
home in the closet. It would be a perfect place to stash
food and drink and keep in the car. She even considered
that maybe she should put it in the trunk, but then thought
that if she needed it, she'd have to ask Mama or Papa to
pull over while she got what she needed. "Better to have it
in the back seat," she thought.*

Taking Trips

Traveling is fun for almost everyone. There is no reason that you cannot travel the world when you have diabetes, but the key to a healthy experience is being prepared. If you take insulin, you may need to talk to your diabetes educator or your doctor beforehand and about trips that cross time lines so that you can keep insulin and meals balanced. There are considerations to be made whether you go east to west or west to east about how your meals are scheduled. Otherwise, the main idea is to always be prepared for both the worst and dumbest things you can imagine, since things often do not go as planned when you are traveling.

Your flight could be cancelled and you may have to spend the night in the airport; you could run out of gas on a long highway in the Midwest; your luggage could go on one plane and you on another; or you could spill your bottle of pills in a foreign town where you don't speak the language. You get the idea: in order to travel safely, you need to expect the unexpected. When traveling, take a prescription or letter from your doctor, stating that you have diabetes, require medication, and carry necessary supplies. If you take insulin, keep it in its original box with the pharmacy label showing, along with a prescription for your syringes. Airlines may search your meter and supplies. Also always wear your medical ID.

Here are some travel tips:

• Take your supplies, rather than thinking you will be able to purchase them where you are going. Some countries have different types and concentrations of insulin, and different ways of measuring in a syringe. Some countries may not have available the diabetes medication that you use, or supplies for your meter.

• Always pack double the supplies that you think you'll need. Also, don't pack them all in one bag. This way, if the bag gets lost or stolen, you still will have some supplies.

• Keep critical supplies, such as medication or insulin, in your carry-on instead of your luggage.

• If you are prone to having low blood sugar, make sure that you always have juice or glucose tablets available.

• Carry a prescription or letter from your doctor stating that you have diabetes and carry syringes with you, if that is the case.

• Find out where you can find diabetes expertise in the areas you are traveling in case of a problem. Have the name and number of a doctor when possible.

• Learn how to say "I have diabetes" in whatever language you need so that you can communicate with a waiter or waitress.

• Carry the number of your home physician with you. In case of questions or problems, you can call for advice if necessary.

• Try requesting a diabetes meal from your airline. Sometimes they are better than the usual trays, and other times not as good. It is usually worth a try!

• If you are on medication or insulin, carry snacks with you so that if a meal is skipped or delayed, you will not become hypoglycemic.

About Substance Abuse (In General)

When you are with your friends, traveling, driving, partying, or just hanging out, you may be tempted to use tobacco, alcohol, or drugs. Obviously, these are not good for anyone, and there are special concerns for people with diabetes who use them. It can be easy these days for teens and adults alike to turn to substances, and they do so for a variety of reasons. Peer pressure, depression, boredom, or a desire to escape reality and be "cool" can all contribute to a teen turning to substances. Sometimes substance use and abuse can go on for a long time before parents or other adults are aware of it. Most teens start by experimenting. They never make a conscious decision, saying, "Okay, I've decided to start using now," but drift into it as they are exposed to the substance, or as people around them are using it. The beginning of substance use can be a slippery slope that slides into substance abuse.

Experimentation can start with curiosity: "What's it like?"

You may wonder what others are talking about and try it out to feel part of the crowd. You may think that you can take it or leave it. It usually doesn't take very much of the substance to get high quickly, and you learn that you can change your mood by its use. As you become more dependent on the substance, you may learn that it helps you do things that you can't do when you're sober, like be more assertive or more social. As a result of using, you may change your circle of friends and may get in trouble with your parents, school, and the law. You find you need more and more of the substance to achieve the same level of being high, and start to believe that the chemical is your "friend." Use becomes abuse as you use the substance in spite of negative consequences. You are hooked.

You become addicted or dependent on the substance. Problems get worse as your life revolves around using. Stable and important people in your life may drop away and you begin to feel guilty, but you can't stop. Your tolerance to the substance increases, and you need more and more of it to reach the same high.

You actually may begin to have blackouts or become sick when using. You try to stop but you can't, and you use substances in larger amounts than you intend. A lot of time is spent being drunk or high. You may be especially at risk for developing a dependency on drugs or alcohol if your parents, grandparents, or brothers and sisters abused alcohol or drugs.

You can see that with any addictive substance, as you become hooked, your priorities and focus shift from the positive things in your life to the use of the substance itself. When you use, it is sometimes hard to believe that the substance is not your friend, but in time, most users are able to see that the substance is the thief that robs you of important things in life! One of the first things you can lose is your health. Diabetes care can become nonexistent as you focus more and more on using and how to get your substance. You may feel physically terrible as you watch your future go into the dumper. It's pretty scary stuff.

If you are finding that you are using or are hooked on an addictive substance, what you should do is both the hardest thing to do and the thing you want to do the least, that is, tell a responsible adult that you are using. It takes courage to ask for help. Most teens also will have the task of dealing with upset parents. It means facing that you are using and may be addicted. But getting help early is the *very best thing that you can do for yourself.* Diabetes and substance use are a bad mix. Let's look more closely at what can happen, depending on what substance you are using.

Bottom Line

Regular use of substances can lead to abuse and addiction. Get help before you slide down the slippery slope.

ABOUT TOBACCO (CIGARETTES AND CHEW)

More teens are smoking and chewing today than any other age group. Often, as in other substance use, it starts with experimentation. The effects of tobacco use are pretty well known, yet pretty well ignored, by young people who smoke. Nicotine is the drug in tobacco that is addictive. You begin using only a small amount, and need more and more as your body begins to tolerate it. Nicotine gives you high blood pressure, since it affects your heart and blood vessels, and this provides a double risk for someone with diabetes. Your kidneys can be destroyed. The smoke from cigarettes causes damage to the little air sacs of your lungs, and can lead to cancer and another disease of the lungs called *emphysema.* People with diabetes who smoke die earlier and are sicker than others.

Some teens choose to chew or use snuff instead of smoking, thinking that it cuts the risk of lung cancer. Chew, however, can cause oral cancer causing irritation to the gums. And the nicotine is absorbed at an even *greater* rate from the mucous membranes of your nose and mouth than by smoking!

If you need help to abstain from smoking or chewing, here

are the top ten reasons I can think of—and they're pretty good ones!

1. Your fingers become stained.
2. Your teeth turn brown.
3. You have smoker's breath.
4. Your clothes smell stale.
5. You can get cancer of the gums, nose, or lungs.
6. You can get high blood pressure.
7. It takes time to find a place to smoke.
8. You can get in trouble with parents, school, or others for smoking.
9. It is expensive.
10. It can lead to diabetes complications.

So, what can you do about smoking?

- If you haven't started smoking, don't!
- If you have started smoking, decide to quit immediately.
- Talk with a health care professional about the best way for you to quit smoking.
- Surround yourself with supportive people. Tell your family and friends that you are quitting and mean it!
- Anticipate challenges, and remember that a lapse can be used as a learning experience.
- Don't give up your efforts to quit!

Bottom Line

It is very smart to choose not to smoke, and it is even smarter not to smoke when you have diabetes.

ABOUT MARIJUANA

People who use pot on a regular basis are more at risk for using other types of drugs and addictive substances. Also, marijuana

---

Bottom Line

If you are using marijuana, drugs, or alcohol regularly, you are headed for trouble. Get help now!

---

often causes an increase in appetite that can definitely be a detriment to any weight control efforts. It can cause you to eat more, nibble, forget how much you have already eaten, and not eat regular healthy meals. In some people, it can cause them to miss meals, which can cause blood sugar to run too low if they take pills or insulin.

Marijuana and other drugs can have effects on blood glucose control. In some cases they may cause blood sugar levels to be too high and in other cases, too low. The chemicals in marijuana can also irritate the mucous membranes in your nose and throat and cause coughing.

Maria's and Tyrone's Story

Tyrone was thinking about grass. He hadn't smoked marijuana and didn't intend to, but it sure was out there. He knew where he could get it in a minute if he wanted to and if he had the money. His friend Jerome used it sometimes—usually on weekends when he was with the gang. Sometimes they offered it to him, but he had always declined. In the fall, it was easy to stay away from it because he usually had a football game. "But frankly," he thought, "I'm just not interested. Seems like a waste of time and money." He knew what Sally was saying about the "slippery slope" because he had a few friends sliding down it now. Jerome was one of them. Tyrone hadn't told his dad yet, but Jerome had just gotten suspended from school for fighting and disrespecting a teacher.

Maria and Rita were also listening. Together they occasionally smoked when they were out. Maria had never bought cigarettes, but had mooched them from other kids.

In some ways, it felt cool and important to smoke. When she smoked she felt both grown up and fake, as though she was trying to be someone she wasn't. But after she had tried it a few times, she didn't like the way her hair and clothing smelled, even the next day. It bothered her that she was hurting her lungs and could get cancer. She knew how easy it was to get hooked on cigarettes. She was afraid to really start smoking for fear that she might not be able to stop. Besides, she didn't have the money anyway. "And Papa would kill me!" she thought. Now that she had diabetes, smoking just didn't seem to be worth the cost.

ABOUT ALCOHOL

Almost everyone knows about the hazards of drinking and driving. "Driving under the influence" is a hazard to your health and everyone else's health. However, almost everyone also knows that many teens either experiment with drinking, or drink regularly. There are the usual concerns about anyone who drinks, and then there are special concerns about a teen who drinks. Drinking alcoholic beverages is illegal for teens because most teens are not mature enough to handle the effects of alcohol responsibly, and it is not a healthy practice.

When you have diabetes, adding alcohol to the picture makes things even more complicated. Alcohol has no nutritional benefit (although there may be some heart and blood vessel benefits to adults who drink red wine or drink very moderately). If you are trying to fit alcohol into a meal plan, know that it is used in a way similar to fat.

Alcohol is processed in the liver and blocks the liver from releasing sugar into the system. If you don't have diabetes, this is usually not a problem. But when you have diabetes, this "block" can be a problem that leads to low blood sugar. There are several problems that can occur when you drink alcohol. Drinking alcohol can cause you to have a low blood sugar, and can be a problem if you take insulin or certain pills. So it is very important that if you have diabetes and are on medication, and you drink alcohol, that you make sure that you also eat.

When you drink, you might not pay attention to the foods you are eating. You might not remember to take your insulin or medication. Plus, alcohol can add extra calories to your diet. One *ounce* of alcohol counts as two fat portions, or about 100 calories! Besides, people with diabetes are also prone to what is known as an "alcohol flush." When they drink alcohol, they may notice that their face gets very red and they feel hot and sweaty.

One question teens often ask is, what do you do when you are at a party or with friends who are drinking? Obviously, one thing you could do would be to say, "No, thank you!" and drink sugar-free soda. Or if it doesn't bother you to talk about it, just say that it is best for you and your diabetes not to drink alcohol.

That's right: It is best for you and your diabetes if you don't drink at all. Plus, it's against the law. However, if you are in a situation where you choose to do so, it pays to be smart about it. (Remember that you do have choices!) Here are some guidelines:

- ➤ Wear your medical ID.
- ➤ Choose light beer, light wine, or white wine instead of liquors. Sweet wines, liqueurs, fruit drinks, or mixed drinks made with regular soda will raise blood glucose levels.
- ➤ Make your own drink so that you know exactly what is in it.
- ➤ Water alcohol down by mixing it with diet soda, club soda, or water.
- ➤ If it is possible, especially with beer, read the label to find out about the amount of carbohydrates.
- ➤ Don't drink on an empty stomach. Plus, drink slowly and sparingly, no more than two drinks.
- ➤ Test your blood glucose before, during, and after drinking.
- ➤ Make sure that you are with someone who knows that you have diabetes and the signs of low blood glucose, if you are on medication.

Bottom Line

The best decision is to choose not to drink. If you do drink, do so carefully, in moderation, and test blood sugar frequently.

Tyrone's Story

Tyrone listened to Sally talk and thought about drinking. He hadn't played around too much with it, but since he was now a junior, a lot of guys were drinking booze. Most of the time it was beer on weekends, and most of the time Tyrone wasn't too involved. Jerome, his best friend, hung out with the drinking crowd and was getting more and more involved. Tyrone hadn't been too comfortable on the nights they were out together. These guys wouldn't take no for an answer and were always pushing him to drink more. Tyrone was even afraid Jerome was headed for trouble. Already his grades were dropping, and he had asked Tyrone last week if he could copy his homework. Tyrone had made a joke and didn't give it to him, but that was unlike Jerome, who was usually on the honor roll. Twice now Tyrone had told those guys to get out of his face. Some of those guys were into some bad stuff. Although he didn't like them much, they got along. He felt that they kind of respected him, probably because of his build and name in football. He thought the drinking was okay, as far as it went, and hadn't ever told his dad. But now, with this new diabetes stuff, he thought, "I just don't know. I don't want to mess anything up. What if I screw up my chance for a scholarship to college?

"On the other hand, what's a few beers gonna do?" He wavered back and forth, caught up in his own thoughts.

Terri called out "Earth to Tyrone . . . Where are you?"

Tyrone smiled, lost in his thoughts, and said nothing. Then Dad spoke up, again making Tyrone surprised at his perception. Sometimes Dad had eyes in the back of his head or something.

"Tyrone's just contemplating how he's gonna stay away from that beer drinking that Jerome and his gang's been offering up. Isn't that right, son? Now, how are you going to do that, son?"

Busted! How did he know? "Um, yeah, Dad. How'd you know?"

"Never you mind how I know. I know a lot of stuff you don't know I know and don't you forget it!"

"Okay. Uh, I guess I've got to find something else to do on Friday nights when Jerome and the gang go out. Dad, I don't want to be drinkin', I really don't. I know that could really mess me up."

"Not to mention the fact that it is illegal! Why don't you go work out at the Y on Fridays? If Jerome won't go with you, take Noah."

Tyrone thought quickly, "Not a bad idea. That will at least get me away from those guys in my face." Noah was not as much fun all the time as Jerome and his gang. But he was decent, a good student, a respectable athlete and they got along. Maybe it would work.

"Okay . . ."

Dad continued, ". . . and other times you are just going to have to learn to say, 'I don't think so!' "

Tyrone figured that it wasn't such a bad idea after all. At least he felt good about his decision to stay away from booze, and was surprisingly relieved that his dad knew about it.

"I don't think so!" Not a bad phrase at all. Tyrone thought that maybe he should practice saying it a bit. He could see in his mind's eye the situation with the guys and Tyrone would just look at them and say, "I don't think so!" He felt more powerful already.

6

Making Choices: For Now, for the Future

We make big and little decisions all day, every day. Sometimes we don't even think much about the little choices we make, and those are most likely not too important in the long run. It may not, ultimately, make a big difference which shirt you wear to school, or which friends you join for lunch. However, the larger decisions might be whether or not to do your homework, apply to colleges, or keep your job. The outcome from these larger decisions has more impact on your life.

The choices you make in your diabetes care probably feel like little decisions. Does it really matter what you eat for breakfast, or whether or not you test your blood sugar? You don't see much immediate outcome from these small decisions. However, this is false thinking. Every time you make a choice that is not in the best interest of your diabetes care, you could be hurting yourself in the long run. It is hard to do or not do something without seeing an immediate effect, but that is exactly what you have to do. Your daily choices affect your long-term health.

Managing Your Diabetes in High School

Obviously, when you have diabetes, there are tasks that you must do to take care of yourself that other kids who don't have diabetes don't have to worry about. It is important that you take care of your diabetes in school, as well as anywhere else that you happen to be. It is your right to be able to do so!

School districts have policies about medications and medical procedures, which are there to keep you and other students safe. Therefore, you, your parents, and the school will need to come together to work out the best possible plan for all concerned. You and your parent(s) should talk about your special needs with a school nurse and other faculty at your school. Your parents will need to call the school and set up a conference. The nurse, teachers, and others in authority positions in the school will need to know about your diabetes needs. Obviously, not everyone in the school needs to know that you have diabetes, but at the very least the school nurse should know. How much and what to tell others depends partially on whether you take medication or insulin, and how prone you might be to have hypoglycemia. (See Chapter 5, When It Comes to Friends and Dating, who to tell.)

After you inform the school, they must evaluate your needs and develop an individualized plan of care as required by federal law. Most of the time, schools are supportive and helpful. They want to help you to take good care of yourself.

The first conference between the school, parents, and student should work out the details of the diabetes plan and how communication will take place. Your parents must be involved in the planning process. One goal is to make the things that you need to do to care for yourself as easy for you as possible in school. Another goal is to keep both you and everyone else safe! Your doctor or diabetes educator will advise you whether or not you will need to do blood glucose tests in school.

It is your right to be able to test your blood sugar as scheduled and at other times, and to have the right foods available to eat. Maybe you won't need to monitor blood during the school day. But if you do, it is important that others be protected from accidentally being stuck on your used lancet. The details about how all of this is to happen need to be worked out.

It is also your right, as a student, to be able to participate fully in all school programs and also to take care of your diabetes. Diabetes should not hold you back from any sport or activity. It should not become an excuse to do or not do anything that is required of other students. There may be times when a schedule change might be in the best interest of your diabetes care, but this should only occur if things cannot be worked out any other way.

Diabetes is considered to be a disability under federal law, and it is against the law for schools to discriminate against someone with a disability. A school staff member must be responsible for making sure that your set plan is followed. That person is usually the school nurse, but not always.

One of the problems in school districts today is that few schools have a full-time nurse. Often one nurse must cover an entire school district and therefore, there might be a secretary or health aide covering emergency needs while the nurse is away. Someone in your school must be designated to cover emergencies. Although this is not usually a big issue for teens with type 2 diabetes, it must be done. Most teens are smart and responsible enough to take care of themselves without difficulty. It is the school's responsibility to allow you to do your diabetes care tasks in the easiest possible way, as long as it is also safe for the other students and staff.

After you figure out who is going to do what and when it will happen, the plan must be written down. This is called an action plan, or an individualized plan of care, which will direct what is to happen and how information will be communicated. See the sample chart.

As a student, it is your responsibility to do what is decided in the plan. You will also need to keep an eye on supplies in the school, and make sure that the school has what they need to help you care for your diabetes. You might need a blood glucose meter and strips to leave in the nurse's office. You also will need to supply syringes, snacks, glucose tablets, or medication when the supply is getting low. Your doctor or diabetes educator will advise you whether or not you will need to do blood glucose tests in school.

Most schools will post a menu ahead of time so that you can see what is being served in the cafeteria and can plan accordingly.

Sample Plan of Care for the Student with Diabetes

Diabetes Care Plan for _____ **(name of student)** _____

School _____

Effective Dates: _____

To be completed by parents/health care team and reviewed with necessary school staff. Copies should be kept in student's classrooms and school records.

Date of Birth: _____ **Grade:** _____
Homeroom Teacher: _____

Contact Information:

Parent/guardian #1: _____
    Address: _____
        Telephone—Home: _____ Work: _____
                Cell Phone: _____

Parent/guardian #2: _____
    Address: _____
        Telephone—Home: _____ Work: _____
                Cell Phone: _____

Student's Doctor/Health Care Provider: _____
    Telephone: _____
  Nurse Educator: _____
    Telephone: _____

Other emergency contact: _____
    Relationship: _____
        Telephone—Home: _____ Work: _____
                Cell Phone: _____

Notify parent/guardian in the following situations: _____
_____
_____

Blood Glucose Monitoring

Target range for blood glucose:
        _____ mg/dl to _____ mg/dl
Type of blood glucose meter student uses: _____
Usual times to test blood glucose: _____

Times to do extra tests (check all that apply):

_____ Before exercise

_____ When student exhibits symptoms of hyperglycemia

_____ After exercise

_____ When student exhibits symptoms of hypoglycemia

_____ Other (explain): _____

_____

Can student perform own blood glucose tests?   Yes   No

Exceptions: _____

School personnel trained to monitor blood glucose level and dates of training: _____

_____

_____

Insulin and/or Medications

Times, types, and dosages of medications to be given during school:

Time	Medication	Dosage
_____	_____	_____
_____	_____	_____
_____	_____	_____

School personnel trained to assist with insulin injection and dates of training: _____

_____

_____

Can student give own injections?   Yes   No

Can student determine correct amount of insulin? Yes   No

Can student draw correct dose of insulin?   Yes   No

For Students with Insulin Pumps:

Type of pump: _____

Insulin/carbohydrate ratio: _____

Correction factor: _____

Is student competent regarding pump?　　　　Yes　No
Can student effectively troubleshoot problems
　　(e.g., ketosis, pump malfunction)?　　　　Yes　No
Comments: _____

_____

_____

Meals and Snacks Eaten at School (The carbohydrate content of the food is important in maintaining a stable blood glucose level.)

	Time	Food content/amount
Breakfast	_____	_____
A.M. snack	_____	_____
Lunch	_____	_____
P.M. snack	_____	_____
Dinner	_____	_____

Snack before exercise?
　　　Yes　　　No　　　_____

Snack after exercise?
　　　Yes　　　No　　　_____

Other times to give snacks and content/amount: _____

_____

A source of glucose, such as _____

_____

should be readily available at all times.
Preferred snack foods: _____

_____

Foods to avoid, if any: _____

_____

Instructions for when food is provided to the class, e.g., as part of a class party or food sampling: _____

_____

_____

Hypoglycemia (Low Blood Sugar)

Usual symptoms of hypoglycemia: _____

_____

_____

Treatment of hypoglycemia: _____

_____

_____

School personnel trained to administer glucagon and dates of training: _____

_____

_____

Glucagon should be given if the student is unconscious, having a seizure (convulsion), or unable to swallow. If required, glucagon should be administered promptly and then 911 (or other emergency assistance) and parents should be called.

Hyperglycemia (High Blood Sugar)

Usual symptoms of hyperglycemia: _____

_____

_____

Treatment of hyperglycemia: _____

_____

_____

Circumstances when urine ketones should be tested: _____

_____

_____

_____

_____

Treatment for ketones: _____

_____

_____

Exercise and Sports

A snack such as _____

_____

should be readily available at the site of exercise or sports.

Restrictions on activity, if any: _____

_____

_____

_____

Student should not exericse if blood glucose is below
_____ mg/dl.

Supplies and Personnel

Location of supplies:

Blood glucose monitoring equipment: _____

_____

_____

Glucagon emergency kit: _____

_____

Snack foods: _____

_____

_____

Medication: _____

_____

_____

_____

_____

_____

Personnel trained in the symptoms and treatment of low and
high blood sugar and dates of training: _____

_____

_____

_____

_____

Signatures

Reviewed by: _____[student's health provider/date]_____

Acknowledged/received by:
_____[guardian/date]_____

Acknowledged/received by:
_____[school representative/date]_____

You may like to buy your lunch most of the time, but when there are days that the lunch meal is not one that is good for you, you may want to pack your lunch.

John is a 16-year-old sophomore in high school who has diabetes, which he controls by watching his diet and exercising. He has done very well staying in control of his blood sugar. When John first got diabetes, he ate the school lunches every day, but it didn't take him too long to figure out that most of the lunches were too high in both fat and carbohydrate. A typical meal was meat loaf, mashed potatoes, rolls, butter, and gravy. Then there was the "gravy train" day. ("Who knows what that is supposed to be, anyhow!") Or there were hot dogs and fries, or macaroni and cheese with a pound of margarine. Yuk! His whole meal plan was sabotaged by lunch! So John, with his mom's help, decided to start packing, and now he only buys lunch if there is something special that he really likes, such as pizza. This plan seems to work for him.

Medication Management in School

If your diabetes is managed by following a program of diet and exercise, your diabetes management in school should not be complicated. However, if you manage your diabetes with pills or insulin, you and the school will also need to work out a plan for taking any necessary shots, how to treat a low blood sugar, and how to test your blood. If you take Metformin (Glucophage) to treat your diabetes and do not take insulin, it is not likely that you will experience low blood glucose. However, other types of pills and insulin can cause a low blood sugar. (See Step #5 in Chapter 2.)

If your doctor recommends that you check blood sugar before lunch, most schools require that you go to the nurse's office, which may involve getting out of class a few minutes early. There should be a plan for the nurse or others who have been designated to help, so that they know what to do if blood sugar is extremely high or extremely low.

Any time that you are feeling signs of low blood sugar (See section 30), it is important that you test your blood sugar and be treated with glucose tablets, juice, and/or crackers. Your teachers and the other school personnel involved with you must be made aware of the signs and understand your needs for treatment.

Since low blood sugar can cause confusion, sleepiness, or disorientation, it is very important to pay attention to these signs, especially if they are happening in school. For example, if your blood sugar is always too low in the class right before lunch, you may not be able to perform well in that class. Don't just put up with it; try to fix the problem by telling your doctor or diabetes educator.

The most likely times for you to become low while in school are:

- During or after gym
- During or after sports
- If you skip a meal or don't eat enough
- If your medication or insulin doses need to be regulated

Your gym teacher and any coaches should be aware that you have diabetes, and be prepared to treat it. If you have friends or a buddy who exercises with you, it is also very smart to let them know what the signs of low blood sugar are, and how to treat it. They may be the first one to pick up on your low blood sugar, if they are with you and know you well. These friends should know how to treat it and where your supplies are kept.

A line of communication should be kept open between you, the school, and your parents. Your parents should know how your diabetes is being managed in school, and if you or the school is having any problems. They can also help by sending a note if you need special care during times of stress or illness.

Erica, a ninth-grader, has had type 2 diabetes for two years. She takes both insulin and metformin and follows her meal plan fairly well. Most of the time her diabetes is in control. However, there were a few days when she had a miserable cold, but went to school anyhow even though her blood sugar was high. Due to high blood sugar, she was extremely thirsty and needed to keep running to the restroom, but two of her teachers refused to let her leave the classroom. Erica was miserable and angry that none of her teachers understood her needs. She realized later that they had not been informed of her special needs and that she might need extra restroom privileges. Her parents then contacted the school nurse, and everything was straightened out.

Missing School

Teens with diabetes should have a normal school attendance record. There is no reason for you to miss any more school than anyone else your age. Sometimes it is tempting to use diabetes as an excuse not to do the things you need to do, but that gains nothing. If blood glucose levels consistently run very high, you may notice that you have less energy than usual. Sometimes it is hard to get out of bed in the morning (but this is generally true for all teens!).

In the first place, there are very few things that you cannot do even if you have diabetes. Second, you should feel good if you have reasonably well-controlled diabetes. If your diabetes control is so poor that it causes you to not feel well enough to go to school, your doctor should be notified. Having a high blood sugar should never keep you from going to school. But having a cold, flu, or viral illness may cause your blood sugar levels to be high and, together with the illness, keep you home. When you are sick, the stress hormones your body makes to fight the illness can make blood glucose levels rise.

By staying home from school, you can make the situation worse. You can start feeling depressed and sorry for yourself. By getting out, getting active, and being with friends, you make a healthier choice than staying home in bed. Also, you don't get behind on schoolwork. Even when you fall off your program, just get up, dust off, and dig in again.

Bottom Line

Don't let diabetes be an excuse.

Tyrone's and Maria's Story

Tyrone thought of his school and the fact that the school nurse was never there. He didn't at first get why it was important that anyone even know that he had diabetes "I mean, so what?" he thought. "It's nobody's business." But then he thought that he really wanted his coach to know, because they were friends anyhow. No one had been more supportive to him than Coach, and it would be good to share this with him. Tyrone thought about how he was going to have to have some other kind of drinks during practice, other than the constant stream of Gatorade, Kool-Aid, and orange juice that he usually drank. Now he was thinking about water or diet soda, with maybe a little bit of Gatorade or juice if he needed it for energy.

Tyrone thought about who else he might tell about his diabetes. Mrs. Leonard, the nurse, should know. "Otherwise," he thought, "no one really needs to know. I'm not taking medication. So as long as I watch my food and exercise, it's nobody's business." Geez, there was a lot to think about.

Maria, on the other hand, was wondering how she would be able to test her blood before lunch. She had already figured out that since she took insulin, it would be best for her to test her blood at lunchtime to see how she was running. Her fourth-period class was on the top floor, the nurse's office on the second, and the cafeteria was in the basement. She really hated to get out of math early to leave, but she hardly had time to eat as it was. Now that she had to go to the nurse's office and test her blood, she didn't know how she'd make it. She turned to Mama and said, "I don't know how I'm gonna do all that!" Mama patted her hand reassuringly and said, "We'll go talk to the school next week and work it out. Maybe you could carry the little meter with you and test in the restroom. We'll see what we can come up with."

Maria didn't think that would work because the school was pretty strict about stuff like that. Her math teacher was pretty nice, however, and he'd probably be understanding. Not only that, she thought, he monitored her study hall in the afternoon, so maybe if she missed anything or had questions she could ask him. Maria felt sort of proud that she had solved that little problem herself!

Thinking About a Career or Job

Kids who grow up in America generally believe that they can be whatever they want to be when they grow up, go wherever they want, and do whatever they please. Is this a dream or a fantasy? Well, in some ways it is fantasy! Although it is wonderful to think that is the case, obviously there are certain limitations that everyone has to deal with when making a decision about the future. For example, not everyone has the brains to become a nuclear physicist. Not everyone has the height to become a good basketball player, and others just don't have the talent to be a professional musician. Each person must take stock of their strengths, weaknesses, talents, and interests before they decide in which direction to head. Of course, there are also people who make no decisions at all but drift afloat in whatever direction the sea of life takes them.

Yet, having goals is a good thing. Maybe college, technical school, or the work force are in your future. But you will need to consider your diabetes when making your decision, along with all of the other obvious considerations.

As you know, diabetes is considered to be a disability. So just as the schools are obligated by federal law to provide for the needs of students with disabilities in the classroom, so are employers responsible for providing reasonable care for the people who work for them. In March 1998, a Federal Court of Appeals ruling determined that the Americans with Disabilities Act protects employees who take insulin on the job. As an employee, you must be given time and provision to take care of your diabetes. This means that if you take insulin and are employed, you must be able to eat properly and on time, test your blood sugar, and take insulin while on the job.

People with disabilities may need to make compromises in life based on what their disability is and what they are able to do. Yet there are inspiring stories of those who have overcome a terrible problem to excel in something. For example, there are people paralyzed from the waist down who make a difference in others' lives by getting up and going to work every day. These cases are inspiring to everyone. Of course, having diabetes is not the same kind of thing as being unable to walk, dress, or feed oneself, although if diabetes complications develop, there are similarities. Still, there are some limitations when you have diabetes, even well-controlled diabetes, regarding certain career choices.

There are restrictions placed on people with diabetes in the military services, and on airline pilots and interstate truck drivers who take insulin. If you want to do one of these jobs, you may want to explore the Internet for the current regulations, because regulations are changing all the time. Until recently there was a ban on people with diabetes scuba diving, but that ban has been lifted. There are also recent changes in the regulations for commercial pilots.

Diabetes is listed in our federal regulations as a disability. It is also a chronic disease. Yet it is a condition where you can lead a relatively "normal" life. The word normal may take on new meaning for you, as it will be normal to follow a meal plan, test blood glucose, exercise, and take medication. But there is very little that you can't do with your life because of diabetes. The idea is not to have your future revolve around diabetes, but rather to fit diabetes into the life that you choose for yourself.

Bottom Line

Fit good diabetes care into the life you choose!

A Time of New Responsibility

What are your responsibilities right now? Homework? Chores? Maybe a job, or trying to get into a college? Add to that list your diabetes. You have a responsibility to take good care of your health. Some teens may not feel that diabetes care is their responsibility, but instead belongs to their parents, doctor, girlfriend, or boyfriend. That thinking has a hole in it. *Each* person is responsible for his or her own health and happiness. No one can do it for you! Your supporters will help you, but no one but *you* is in charge.

High school is the time to begin to take on responsibility for yourself. Some teens start taking on responsibility even earlier than that. You may be used to your parents doing it all for you, and parents can continue to hang in there with those tasks, not wanting to give them up. Of course, your parents are concerned for you and your health and might be afraid you will not be safe if they don't do things for you.

Parents fear that you might not take care of yourself. That is understandable, because your parents love you, and want you to be healthy. The answer to the independence tug-of-war is for you to show that you are trustworthy. Show your parents that you are interested and willing to take care of yourself and that you will do a good job. When your parents are convinced that you can do the job yourself as well, if not better, than they have done it for you, they can back off and relax, allowing you to take the responsibility.

You can start to prove your self-responsibility in a lot of ways.

➤ Test blood sugar when you are supposed to without being asked.

➤ Record blood sugar tests.

➤ Look for patterns of high or low blood sugar levels and talk to your parents about how to solve the problem.

➤ Be assertive about managing your schedule so that you can take care of diabetes.

➤ Talk to your parents about how to improve your diabetes care.

➤ Remember your doctor appointments, remind your parents about them, and make sure that you have transportation to them.

➤ Answer the questions at your appointment, and ask a few of your own.

➤ Make sure that you have supplies available long before they run out. Don't wait until the last minute before telling your parents.

➤ If you drive, make sure that you do what is necessary while on the road to care for your diabetes. If you take insulin, make sure that you always test your blood sugar before driving.

➤ Teach your friends about your diabetes care tasks.

➤ Avoid tobacco, alcohol, and other addictive substances.

➤ Wear a medical ID.

Wearing Medical ID

You may feel that wearing a medical ID is like advertising to the world that you have diabetes. Not true! People wear IDs for many reasons, such as food allergies, contact lenses, asthma, heart conditions, or bee sting allergies. Some people even list their medications on the ID.

Okay, so you may never need one. That is the hope, but if you haven't yet gotten the concept that when you have diabetes you need to be prepared for the unexpected, now is the time to think about it. Your medical ID is not an advertisement, but a safety net. If you were ever in a serious accident or became unconscious, medical personnel would be able to give you proper care if they knew you have diabetes.

There are a whole variety of different types of IDs. You can get a neck chain, bracelet, or ankle chain, and they come in materials such as nylon, stainless steel, gold fill, or gold. There are types that clip on a watch, and cute charms. Ask your diabetes educator to show you samples of various types of ID. It is smart to wear an ID and also to carry a card in your wallet with emergency information.

Some sources for Medical IDs are:

Medic Alert Foundation U.S.
2323 Colorado Ave.
P.O. Box 1009
Turlock, CA 95382-9009
1-800-432-5378

Life Alert
P.O. Box 68527
Portland, OR 97268
1-403-258-0822

Goldware
P.O. Box 22335
San Diego, CA 92192
1-800-669-7311
www.goldware-ID.com

Miss Brooks Co. (charms for children and teens)
P.O. Box 558
Bryant, AK 72089
1-888-417-7591

Diabetes Research and Wellness Foundation
1206 Potomac St., NW
Washington, DC, 20007
1-202-298-9211
www.diabeteswellness.net

American Medical Identifications Inc.
P.O. Box 925617
Houston, TX 77292-5617
1-713-695-7358

Adult Choice: Connecting with a New Health Care Team

Because children and teens with diabetes have their own unique problems, they usually do best when they are followed in a major medical center that has a diabetes care team. Pediatric diabetes centers are equipped to follow teens through their graduation from high school; many, but not all, will continue treating young adults beyond that. Some teens are completely comfortable with going to a pediatric diabetes center, and others may feel too old and uncomfortable when they are there with a bunch of toddlers and little kids. Some places, however, do not have diabetes teams available; in such an instance, it will be important to choose a doctor, diabetes educator, and dietitian.

Since type 2 diabetes used to be called "maturity" or "adult-onset" diabetes, some people feel that since teens with type 2 have the "adult" form of the disease, it doesn't matter whether or not a doctor who sees only adults should follow them. However, teens have their own issues separate from adults, and should go somewhere where the medical care is experienced and suitable for the special needs of teens. Adolescent medicine is its own specialty, and teens with diabetes are no exception. Take a moment right now and think about what feels right for you.

Independence brings on new responsibilities that will need your attention, and one of these responsibilities involves taking charge of your own health care needs. As you grow up and move from pediatric to adult healthcare, a new task may be finding a new doctor near your new school, or finding a new health care team to monitor your diabetes as you become an adult. One of the worst things that can happen during this transition is for you to put off finding a new health care team and so end up ignoring your diabetes. That's bad news! Emergency treatment then can be like putting a Band-Aid on a broken back: It won't make a difference.

It is easy to make your job, school, friends, TV, sports, or other activities a priority in your life. It is common for any or all of these activities to get in the way of diabetes care, but ignoring diabetes care isn't the answer. It doesn't make sense to ignore your diabetes, when ultimately diabetes complications could prevent you from doing the very thing that you want to do!

When people don't have health care, their diabetes suffers. If you don't have a doctor or connect with a health care team, it is hard to stay motivated to take care of your diabetes. One of the jobs of diabetes educators, dietitians, psychologists, and social workers is to help to keep you on track. It isn't surprising that teens and young adults who have a history of missed appointments also have a poor track record in sticking with their program. These teens are most likely to have poor blood glucose control and to have, ultimately, complications of diabetes.

However, sometimes when you make the transition from child care to adult care, it can be a rude awakening! Pediatric centers that specialize in teen and adult care can nurture you in a way you do not find in adult care. You may miss the gentle nudges and encouragement in the right direction; most adult care settings do not have a similar approach. Most adult care centers have an expectation that you will take responsibility for your own care. One teen put it this way:

When I was a teenager, my mother always set up the appointments and drove me there. She did all of the talking and knew everyone. The staff got me to go to camp, become a counselor, and come to some support groups. One of the nurses actually called me weekly to see how I was doing when I went through a period when things weren't going so well. They sort of pulled me along and somehow sent me in the right direction. I didn't really appreciate it, though, because I thought it would always be like that.

It was a rude awakening when I went to my first adult clinic. First of all, I think because everyone is new and you don't have a history with people, it feels strange. Everyone was in a big hurry. The appointments were too fast and there wasn't time to talk. By the time I got around to thinking about my questions, the appointment was over. Although everyone was nice, and they were encouraging, I didn't feel like they really cared whether I did stuff or not. I suddenly realized that I am the one in charge who has to take care of myself. No one else really cares, except for my family and friends, of course, whether I do it or not. No one is going to beg me or push me. It's all up to me! What a smack of reality that was!

Such changes can be hard to deal with. Sometimes it is smart to not make too many changes at one time. Maybe you don't need to adjust to college and a new doctor all at one time. Perhaps you could find a doctor close to school to see you while you are there, but continue to see your usual team when you are home for the summer or holidays for the first year or so. There are all sorts of ways to work it out, depending on where you are and who is available to you.

Bottom Line

Stay connected to a health care team!

Getting the Most Out of Your Health Care Visits

When you visit your team members, it is smart to be prepared so that you can get the most out of your visits. (Remember, your parents and/or your insurance company or coverage is paying for your diabetes visits, so you might as well take advantage of it!) Here are some things to think about when you visit your health care team:

• *Be prepared:* Find out exactly where to go, what time to go, and whether or not you will need to have blood drawn before your appointment. Take your blood glucose meter, strips, medical records, prescriptions, and records of blood sugar numbers. Your doctor may also want a urine sample. Write down a list of questions and prescriptions that you need so that you don't forget to ask what you want to know while you're there. Your doctor will also want to know the dates and brief details of anything unusual that has happened since your last visit, including illness, surgery, trauma, and medications taken.

• *Speak up:* Whatever your issues and questions are, get them off your chest right away. Don't wait until the end of your appointment, when time has run out, to discuss your concerns.

• *Be honest:* If a member of your team has expectations that you think you'll never be able to meet, it is much better to tell them than to go home and never do it at all. For example, if someone suggests that you go home from school and jog every day from 4:30 to 5:00, and you have a problem with that, don't hesitate to say, "Well, I really don't think that will work. I know myself, and I'm really tired when I come home, and besides, two days a week I don't get home until six o'clock, anyhow."

• *Offer solutions:* As the center of the team, you certainly can have some input into the way things are going. If you don't know what the goal is, *ask!* If you do know that the goal is, for example, to exercise every day, you might say, "Well, I know that the 4:30 P.M. jogging plan is never going to work, but I probably could do twenty minutes on a bike right after dinner."

Let's face it, most of us don't like to go to doctors. It takes time and money, and when you go, you have to face your problems. Sometimes people don't like to go because they don't want to hear what the doctor has to say, or don't want to find out that they have to do some things they might not feel like doing. But, again, that old ostrich-stick-your-head-in-the-sand approach is not going to help. Sometimes teens even fight with their parents about going to the doctors. But Mom or Dad are simply doing what they're supposed to be doing as good parents when they make you go. They are taking care of you and being responsible for your health until you are old enough, and responsible enough, to do it for yourself. They do it because they love you. When you're an adult, it's up to *you* to do what you can to help yourself stay healthy. The American Diabetes Association recommends that you visit your doctor every three months.

> ### Bottom Line
> You deserve good care. Be your own advocate.

Hanging in There with Your Diabetes Program

You will learn as you go that some things that have to do with your diabetes care are negotiable and some are not. For example, seeing your doctor every three months should not be negotiable. Other things that aren't negotiable are taking your medicine in the right dose and on time. Other things may take more judgment, such as how much and what foods to eat. Sometimes you might make better decisions than others.

Jim, a 15-year-old with type 2 diabetes for over two years, did really well at first, then did poorly, then really well, then not so well. The problem, as he described it, was that he was an "all-or-nothing" kind of guy. He was either on top of his program, doing it all and doing it well, or he did none of it. When he fell off his program, he would get angry at himself, get discouraged, and quit. Then when things got really bad and he felt physically horrible, he'd get back on his program for a while. Jim could have used a more reasonable and steady approach. Sometimes he was trying so hard to be perfect at everything that he burned out! In any case, he should never give up completely. For example, sometimes he surrendered to the allure of pie and ice cream. But instead of throwing in the towel and saying, "I blew it and now it's ruined! I quit," he could say "Okay, I fell off my program, but this is a new day!" and continue where he left off.

MANAGING THE STRESSFUL TIMES IN YOUR LIFE

When you are stressed out about something or your body is under physical stress, your diabetes control might suffer. First of all, being stressed causes the release of the hormone epinephrine, which has the effect of raising blood sugar levels. So when you are stressed, your blood sugar may run higher than usual. Also, when something stressful is going on in life, it is common to let things go.

Have you figured out that when something stressful happens, that seems to be the exact time that you lose your keys, forget things, or are otherwise distracted? What is unique about stress is that it is completely individual. What stresses one person may not stress another at all. Do you know kids who never get disturbed about exams, yet absolutely fall apart when their girlfriend or boyfriend breaks up with them? Someone else may be a complete basket case during finals, but handle a lack of sleep just fine.

As you've read, what happens when you are under stress is that your adrenal glands make adrenaline (epinephrine), which is the same hormone that is made to raise blood sugar if blood sugar levels are low (see Chapter 2). The adrenaline then will send blood sugar levels up.

Of course, there are different kinds of stress and different levels of intensity, and you cannot predict how your body will respond. For example, brief stressors might be losing homework, taking a test, or having a fight with your sister. These are minor problems that could happen every day, and most likely will not have a big negative impact on your blood glucose control. On the other hand, having family problems, having a parent who is alcoholic, having a death in the family, watching your parents go through a divorce, or seeing something violent can cause sustained stress and poor blood sugar control. Or physical stress coming from an illness such as a cold, flu, viral illness, or injury, can make your blood sugar rise.

The other thing that happens when there is stress in your life is that you may find you don't take good care of yourself. Other things become a priority, and diabetes care suffers. The thing is, we don't live life in a bubble. You can't protect yourself from having stress in your life. But if you find that life is always too big a mess for you to do the things you need to do and that your diabetes care is poor, you will need to figure out what to do about it. A social worker or therapist may be able to help.

One thing that is important to remember during times of major stress is that there are some basic minimum survival rules. These will not promote best blood sugar control, but if you at least do the minimum, you should be safe until you can get back on track.

Minimum Survival Tasks:

➤ Always take your medication.
➤ Test blood sugar levels when you can.
➤ Don't skip meals.

What can be very helpful in easing stress is to determine what it is that is stressing you. Often you may know what that is, and other times, you might not. Maybe it is a whole bunch of things, or maybe it is only one situation or person. Then you will need to figure out what to do to handle it. In other words, you will need a stressbuster!

If you have a physical illness, there really isn't a whole lot you can do about it. And the small things that happen every day are probably just going to happen. But perhaps you know that you relax when you exercise, walk, or listen to music. Exercise is a great stressbuster, and it kills a whole bunch of birds with one stone. When you exercise, you unwind and relieve stress, lower your blood sugar, *and* burn calories. On the other hand, maybe an hour vegging in front of the TV will help. Or try laughing with a friend, seeing a comedy movie, or maybe getting at your homework so that you don't have to worry about it. If you try to relax and can't do so because your problems feel really big, perhaps you will need a counselor or another person to talk to.

7

Finding Help When You Need It

Knowing When to Call for Help

Knowing when to call for help is an important piece of information. When there is an emergency, everyone seems to know that they should call 911. But when you have diabetes, sometimes it is not that clear when and who to call.

First off, when you are sick, vomiting, or have diarrhea, it is important that you call your doctor. You will need to know what to do with your diabetes medications or insulin. Many people mistakenly think that if they are throwing up, they will not need to take insulin. Usually what happens, however, is that when you are sick, the stress of the illness and the adrenaline that is pumped out from it cause blood sugar levels to go up. Sometimes, even though you are not eating, you may need more insulin than usual! If you become very sick with a fever or flu, it is very important to stay hydrated by drinking as much as you can, and to also keep checking blood sugar levels frequently. If you can't hold food or beverages in your stomach, the first thing to do is to try to settle your stomach. Sometimes flat soda (regular not diet) will work, or a Popsicle or some hard candy. This is not the time to worry about not eating sugar, but let your blood sugar tests be your guide. If your blood sugar is high, it does not make a lot of sense to drive it even higher. If you can't stop vomiting, call your doctor immediately, as you might need some IV fluids.

Guidelines for When to Call Your Doctor

- Blood sugar levels that remain over 200 for more than a few days.
- Illness such as fever, vomiting, or diarrhea
- Any sign of infection, including redness, pus, drainage, pain, fever or swelling
- Repeated or unexplained low blood sugar
- Physical concerns that are persistent or disabling
- Signs of drinking a lot, voiding a lot, or unexplained weight loss

Resources

There are all kinds of places where you can get more information on diabetes. Some of the publications are listed below, along with organizations that are helpful. It is always a good thing to find other people who are dealing with the same issues you are because not only do you hear through the grapevine about new products, technology, research, and care, but when you hear how others cope with their diabetes, it can also give you some new thoughts about dealing with it. There are all sorts of support groups and organizations out there that will give you information and help. You might ask your diabetes educator if there are any teen groups in your area. Another great way of meeting others is at diabetes camp. Camp is a place where good friendships are formed. Also, you might benefit from joining an organization in your area where you have an interest and might even volunteer your time. Here are some places where you can find help and information on diabetes.

American Association of Diabetes Educators—to get the name of a Certified Diabetes Educator in your area call 1-800-832-6874 *www.aadenet.org/*

American Diabetes Association
1-800-Diabetes
www.diabetes.org

American Dietetic Association
1-800-366-1655
www.eatright.org.

American Heart Association
1-800-242-8721
www.americanheart.org.

Calorie Control Council
1-404-252-3662
www.caloriecontrol.org.

American Podiatric Medical Association
1-800-FOOTCARE
www.apma.org

Disability Rights Education and Defense Fund, Inc.
1-800-466-4232
dredfca@AOL.com

Equal Employment Opportunity Commission
1801 L. Street, NW
Washington, DC 20507

International Diabetic Athletes Association
1-800-898-IDAA
www.getnet.com/~idaa/

International Diabetes Federation for information about diabetes
in other countries
Rue Defacqz 1, β-1000
Brussels, Belgium 32-2/538-5511
www.idf.org

Juvenile Diabetes Foundation International
1-800-553-2873
www.jdfcure.org

The National Diabetes Education Program—This is a joint program of the National Institutes of Health and the Centers for Disease Control and Prevention. Its purpose is to improve treatments and outcomes for people with diabetes.
1-800-438-5383
www.niddk.nih.gov/health/diabetes/nedp/ndep.htm

National Diabetes Information Clearinghouse
One Information Way
Bethesda, MD 20892-3560
1-301-654-3327
www.niddk.nih.gov/health/diabetes/ndic.htm
This site has all kinds of diabetes information. Send for the free publications "Diabetes in African Americans," "Employment, Discrimination and Diabetes," or "Building Understanding to Prevent and Control Diabetes Among Hispanics/Latinos," if you are interested.

National Eye Institute
1-301-496-5248
www.nei.nih.gov

National Information Center for Children and Youth with Disabilities
P.O. Box 1492
Washington, DC 20013-1492
1-800-695-0285
www.aed.org/nichcy

National Kidney Foundation
30 E. 33rd St.
New York, NY 10016
1-800-622-9010
www.kidney.org

Prevent Blindness America
500 E. Remington Rd.
Schaumburg, IL 60173

1-800-331-2020
www.preventblindness.org

OTHER RESOURCES

Children with diabetes website at:
www.childrenwith diabetes.com.

Countdown (a quarterly magazine on diabetes research, particularly focused on youth)
Juvenile Diabetes Foundation International
432 Park Ave. South
New York, NY 10016
1-800-223-1138

Diabetes Interview (a monthly newspaper with diabetes-related news, including diabetes research and products)
Published by Kings Publishing
3715 Balboa St.
San Fransciso, CA 94121
1-415-387-4002

Diabetes in Control Newsletter (a weekly on-line newsletter)
www.diabetesincontrol.com

Diabetes Forecast (a monthly magazine)
Published by American Diabetes Association, Inc.
National Service Center
1660 Duke St.
Alexandria, VA 22314
1-800-232-3472

Diabetes Self-Management (bimonthly magazine)
Published by R.A. Rapport Publishing, Inc.
150 West 22nd St.
New York, NY 10011
1-800-234-0923

Maria's and Tyrone's Story

Their time with Sally was ending, and they felt fairly confident that they would know what to do. Maria's Mama, however, said it felt a little bit like taking a new baby home from the hospital: There was a lot to do and a lot to think about, and she didn't want to make any mistakes. Sally assured them that it would be hard to make a mistake that would be life-threatening, and if they made small mistakes, well, they'd just learn from them.

Tyrone and Maria traded e-mail addresses so they could check to see how each other was doing once in a while. Sally wished them good luck and good-bye, and said she'd be available to answer their questions in the future.

8

Real Thoughts from Real Teens

When I started to write this book, I told some of my patients about it with the aim of picking their brains to see what they thought would be effective, readable, and interesting for them. I asked if they would read a book on diabetes, and if they'd be interested in talking about their own experiences. As is the case in most situations, many more teens said that yes, they'd like to participate, than actually were able to follow through, but a few very dedicated and interested teens offered to answer questions and comment on their struggles with diabetes. I thank them for their participation, honesty, and candor.

This chapter is for and about them, and reflects the comments of teens with type 2 diabetes in the real world today and how they deal with some aspects of their own diabetes. I hope that their comments help you to think about the issues of diabetes, and let you know that you are not alone in dealing with them.

The Teen Commentators

Aloin—an African-American 15-year-old male who was diagnosed with type 2 diabetes at age 15. He is currently controlling his diabetes with diet only.

Bridget—a 16-year-old Caucasian female who was diagnosed at age 15. She currently treats her diabetes with Glucophage (metformin) and Precose.

Justin—a 15-year-old Caucasian male who was diagnosed at age 13. He currently treats his diabetes with insulin and Glucophage.

Kelsie—an 18-year-old Caucasian female who was diagnosed with type 2 diabetes at the age of 14. She currently treats her diabetes with Glucophage.

Jean (Interviewer)—*I'd like for you to share things that you don't hear from your health care professional that might be helpful for another teen with type 2 diabetes. I would like to hear the hard parts, what you have learned, and what solutions you may have come up with to handle problems. Because part of this book talks about beginning to learn to solve diabetes problems yourself, I am interested to hear how you choose to cope with things.*

One of the first questions I have is about the time when you first got diabetes. I'd like to hear what you thought about it and how it went for you.

Kelsie: My mom wanted me to lose weight, and that is why she first put me in a study. I didn't know what was going on, and my doctor then asked me to be in a study on type 1 diabetes. But it turned out that I had type 2 diabetes. When I first got it I was scared.

Aloin: Well, I've had diabetes for about 2 years. I got it when I was on vacation with my family in Florida. I was drinking about every 4 seconds, and had to go to the bathroom a lot. I had sugar in my urine. I was on insulin for the first couple of weeks. I didn't like that at all. Then we came back home and I've been here dealing with it ever since.

What did you think about diabetes?

Kelsie: I didn't know what it meant, really. I still don't!

Aloin: I knew a little bit about it because my Grandma's on insulin. I think I have a pretty good understanding.

Learning about diabetes is so important! Here we have one person who has diabetes, who has been through a diabetes education program, and still *doesn't understand what it is! And we have someone else who feels pretty secure in his understanding. If you don't feel that you have a good understanding, talk to a doctor or your diabetes educator and begin reading.*

How do you think you take care of yourself?

Kelsie: Well, actually, I'm not too good at that. I think that the only thing I need to do is to lose weight. I try but it is hard.

Aloin: I try to get my weight down, so I won't have to go back on insulin.

Justin: I really don't like to take two shots of insulin every day.

Bridget: I try, but I really don't like that I have to work so hard to lose weight. Sometimes it feels like I'm hardly eating anything compared to what some of my friends eat!

What is the hardest part of having diabetes for you?

Justin: The hardest part is having to watch everything I eat while others eat what they please. It's also hard to have to handle those two shots of insulin a day.

Kelsie: I hate it that I can't eat what other people eat. Not eating the candy and stuff really is the hardest.

Aloin: Watching a diet is hard. I follow it sometimes, but I'm still just a little bit overweight.

Bridget: I follow my meal plan pretty well because I want to lose the weight, but it is hard to do. It's hard to be out with friends when they get stuff that you can't have.

Well, it sounds as though all of you find following a meal plan and losing weight to be the hardest part. I'm not surprised, but here you are, a teen who now has to cut calories, be careful about food, and lose weight. How do you deal with that when some amazing kind of food is around?

Justin: Well, sometimes, if it's something I want, I will take just a little of something offered, or I'll bring along a healthy treat for me. That helps, for the most part.

Kelsie: I don't deal with it very well. If I want it, I eat the whole thing.

Bridget: I sometimes go off my meal plan. That makes me depressed. I feel like I'm doing something wrong or something.

Aloin: I try to just watch and be careful, but sometimes I don't do it. I only have a little bit of weight to lose. Sometimes when I eat something, I then go out and play basketball. I'll tell you what works for me: the idea of having to go back on insulin shots. I'll do *anything* to avoid that.

It seems as though everyone is motivated by something different. Justin is motivated to care for himself because he hopes to not take insulin someday. Bridget is motivated by weight control. Aloin has a pretty healthy approach, as he tries to satisfy himself yet still be in control, and he exercises then when he needs to. Kelsie, on the other hand, openly admits that she doesn't even try to do what she needs to do for herself.

Although diabetes is not usually funny, sometimes funny things happen. I think it is important not to lose your sense of humor about things. Do you have any funny stories, or has anything amusing happened regarding your diabetes that you could tell us?

Justin: No.

Kelsie: There's not too much that's been funny.

Bridget: It's no joke. It's life!

Aloin: I can't think of anything funny, but I do think you should try to have fun with it!

Sometimes you just have to laugh. This is actually kind of gross, but one time a while back when my kids were younger, I was cooking dinner and stopped to test my blood sugar. I didn't know I was still bleeding as I walked around the kitchen touch-

ing things, cooking, and stirring. When my son walked into the kitchen he looked at the floor, the counter top, the cutting board, the fridge, and the stove, and thought I had been killed or something. There was blood everywhere!

Bridget: Yeah, did you ever do a finger prick and squeeze and the blood squirted out three different holes?

It's important to continue to look for the humor in things!

What is the most helpful thing that your parents and friends do to help you take care of yourself?

Justin: Well, one thing they do is make sure that they have foods or snacks that are lower in sugar so I can share in the fun at parties or family dinners.

Aloin: My parents care about me and I know it. So I try to listen to them.

Kelsie: My mom helps me. I also have a friend whose mom knows that I have diabetes, and when I'm over there she makes sure that I eat the right foods. Sometimes they do eat junk, and when I'm there she puts it away because I can't have it. That's nice.

Bridget: Sometimes it is hard when people eat things right in front of you that you want and you know you can't have. I have my own drawer of things I can have in the kitchen, so when my family is eating something I can't, I don't feel as left out.

So you find that other people who are considerate of your needs help you by making it easy for you to stay on your program. That's good. But now let's talk about the other side of this. What is least *helpful to you in your diabetes care?*

Justin: I don't find it very helpful when people are always saying, "Don't eat this, don't eat that." They do it more than is necessary. *I* know what not to eat. Sometimes it makes me so mad that it makes me want to eat the wrong things. But then I remember how sick I was before and I really don't want to ever do that again.

Kelsie: I said that my mom helps me and she does. But she also nags and that isn't helpful. She tells me what I can or can't eat all the time. She worries and sometimes will hide stuff. But I usually know where it is or can find it if I want to.

Bridget: My mom and dad are really helpful to me and I appreciate it, but I don't like it when they worry and fuss. It's like they don't trust that I'll do the right thing to take care of myself.

Do you feel as though you are doing a good job dealing with your diabetes?

Aloin: Yes, I do think I'm doing a good job. My last HbAlc was normal and I'm only a little bit overweight. I probably don't follow my diet exactly. I forget how many calories I'm supposed to be on. I think somewhere around 2,000 calories. I don't eat lunch right now, but at the beginning of the year, I bought lunch. I eat yogurt and pretzels sometime for lunch. That's probably not what I'm supposed to be doing, but it seems to be working. I don't really have an exercise program, either, but I do try to get as much exercise as I can. I like to shoot hoops and play a lot of basketball.

Justin: I think I do a good job, too. I try to watch what I eat and most of the time my sugar is good. Getting my weight down is another story. But I keep trying and won't give up.

Kelsie: I think I do a good job because I have good cholesterol and good blood test numbers. The only thing the matter with me is that I have diabetes.

Is there anything about diabetes that scares you?

Kelsie: I know about complications and do think about them sometimes. I think it's really scary that complications could happen to you. You could die. That's a pretty hard thing to have to deal with.

Aloin: Complications don't bother me. I'm doing okay. In fact, I don't know that I could do any better. I think it will just be fine. You can't let it get you down.

Bridget: I think that complications are depressing, but I try not to think about it. I'm doing okay and feel healthy. You just can't let it get in your way.

How do your friends handle your diabetes?

Kelsie: My friends are fine with it. I like to dance a lot, and I know I should have exercise, so I dance in my room and outside with my friends. And I told you about my friend who is really helpful.

Bridget: Well, if they are a true friend, they will help you. When you go out to eat, they don't throw stuff you can't have in your face.

Aloin: My friends are all okay with it. Most of them know, and it's no big deal. They don't mess with me and I do my own thing.

If you could tell a newly diagnosed teen with type 2 diabetes one or two important things that you have learned along the way, what would they be?

Justin: Try to remember to check your glucose level often so you can be sure you are eating correctly. Remember that the shots are helping to keep you well.

Kelsie: Eat the right foods, because if you don't, bad things can happen to you.

Aloin: Just listen to your parents. Don't let it get you down, try your best with it, and don't give up easily. Try to have fun along the way.

Bridget: Take your medicine on time! Study your blood sugar records for patterns of highs and lows, and make smart choices in your diet, like choosing baked chips instead of fried.

It isn't surprising, of course, that you are all struggling with some of the same issues: weight loss, watching your diet, getting exercise, taking medication, etc. It is hard to live with, and it does not go away. Part of the hard part is that you cannot say that if you do this thing or that thing, your diabetes will be cured

and stay that way. It is the uncertainty of what is going to happen that can be very hard to deal with.

I liked that you were able to generally agree that nagging
parents, friends, and relatives are not helpful to keeping you on
course, but that friends who understand and respect your need
to stay on your program are helpful.

I'm still waiting for you to think of things that are funny about
diabetes. I believe that it is so important to keep your sense of
humor and try to see the humor in life. Sometimes the strangest
things happen, and I think to myself that God must have a sense
of humor! Laughter IS good medicine, and it will help reduce
your stress, keep you positive, and when you can laugh at yourself, you often deal with negative things better. So keep smiling!

Lastly, you are all saying, "Don't give up! Hang in there! Do
what you gotta do and it will be okay." That message will be
quite helpful to newly diagnosed teens with diabetes who are
scared, confused, and lost. Just to know that you are doing this
and are doing well with it ought to be very helpful to them.

9

For Parents: What Your Teen Wishes You Understood

Most parents have heard their kids say to them, "You just don't understand!" It *is* sometimes difficult to understand what our children must deal with, and sometimes when we think we understand, we really don't. The problems that our youth have today have never been present to the same degree in prior generations.

However, in spite of all the difficulties that youth in our culture face, most teens want the love and approval of their parents. Sometimes they may not know how to express it, and may test you a lot to see how far they can stretch, but they ultimately desire a close relationship with their parents. It has been shown in research that teens who stay out of trouble most often do so because of a strong relationship with a parent.

I've talked to many teens with type 2 diabetes, and there are lots of things they wish you could understand about them. Unless you have diabetes yourself, she probably doesn't think that you understand what it is like to have to deal with watching a diet, having to exercise, and sticking your finger. She wants you to know that she doesn't want to feel different from her friends. She doesn't like having to test her blood sugar in front of everyone, yet doesn't like to have to leave her friends to test her blood.

Neither does she like having to follow a meal plan. She misses having the freedom to eat what she pleases. Also, she hates it when people presume she can't eat things she actually can have, and they don't even offer them to her. She may say that it doesn't bother her when others eat candy bars or brownies in front of her, but it does.

She also feels that she is expected not to want something she does want. When her siblings eat chips and cookies, sometimes her discipline crumbles. But neither does she want her siblings to resent her because they are not allowed to have candy and snacks in the house because of her diabetes. The fact that this is not a "diet" but a lifetime meal plan sometimes makes her cry.

If she is overweight, she wants you to know how lousy it feels to be heavier than her friends, and sometimes ridiculed by her peers for being so. She wants to hear from you that if she works hard to follow her meal plan, she can lose the weight and be healthy. She wants you to believe in her and help her with it. She does not want to hear negative things about being overweight nor derogatory comments about her weight. She wants encouragement and role modeling from you on how to eat right and exercise. The discipline you show in your life sets an example for her to follow.

Your teen will want you to allow him to handle his diabetes in his own way, as long as he is being responsible in caring for himself. He may want to tell friends and others about diabetes himself, or not. He probably will want you to withhold announcements about diabetes to others, such as to the waitress and others seated at the table, or whoever is within earshot. There may be instances, however, when he'd like you to ease his way by helping him tell others. He'll tell you when these times are, but most of the time he'd prefer to tell others himself.

He gets furious when you remind him to test his blood sugar or record the number in a log, yet he cannot seem to remember to do it himself. He doesn't want you to be involved in his diabetes care because he wants to be independent. He wants to do it himself and wants you to know that you can trust him, yet he can't seem to always follow through.

He knows that sometimes he slips up on his testing, or eats extra food, but doesn't want you to be worried or angry with him when he has high numbers. Sometimes he knows why his numbers are high (because he ate too much, or a sweet food), and sometimes he has no idea why his blood sugar numbers are high. When you get upset, worried, or "freaked out" when numbers are high, it becomes tempting for your teen to hide the number, falsify the number, or quit testing. He'd like to be honest about it, but doesn't want to worry you any more than he already has. And he doesn't want more nagging than already goes on. Sometimes, it's just easier to play "Let's not, and say we did."

Frequently other things get in the way of the things he intends to do. In spite of the fact that he pushes you away, he really relies on your power and protection. He needs to know that you will protect him from himself, if need be. He needs to know that you care and will be involved in his care, no matter what he says and does. He actually feels very scared when he thinks about being completely at the mercy of his own self-control and self-discipline.

If your teen takes insulin, she wants you to understand what an enormous inconvenience it is. She now has to take insulin wherever she goes, in case she goes out for dinner. Although most of her friends are supportive, she doesn't like the attention she gets when she has to take a shot. Having to keep insulin cool, and carry it to school or afterschool activities, is a "big pain." She'd like to take and carry her insulin as discretely as possible. Of course, there are also hypoglycemia and glucagon to have to deal with in school, activities, and field trips. Some of her teachers handle the information about low blood sugar just fine, and others became "all anxious" about it. She doesn't like to feel low and have to eat something in the middle of class with everybody watching her. Neither does she like to have to leave class and go to the nurse's office, because she misses what goes on in the classroom. Besides that, it is disrupting. And she really is unhappy when other people fuss over her when she is feeling hypoglycemic. Your teen might like to have your help in dealing with the school and others, but may not desire parental intrusion on her turf.

Your teen wants you to know that diabetes has placed a scary burden on her life. She had never before thought of being sick or dying, and now she has a disease that suggests she could have frightening complications unless she follows her program. She's doing the best she can, and doesn't want to be sick now or in the future. She wonders how she is supposed to balance all the things that are important to you and herself, such as homework, job, and other activities, *and* keep diabetes a priority. Those other things used to have top priority, and she is told that diabetes shouldn't interfere with anything she wants to do with life, yet how can she do it all? She may need help in prioritizing and fitting her diabetes tasks into her normal routine. She wonders how much she can deviate from her program and yet stay well. Is she expected to stick with it 100 percent of the time? Is 90 percent good enough? How about 50 percent? How much can she "get away with," i.e., go off her management plan, and stay healthy? In fact, maybe she'll push until she finds out. Anything bad that might happen, such as complications, is probably a long way off: "I'll deal with that later. By that time, they might have a cure!"

Parenting a Teenager: What a Job!

As a parent of a teen, you most likely know all too well the rigors of your parenting job. The behaviors of teens are well known and universal. Raising your child into adulthood is one of the most important and difficult things you will ever do. When parents talk about life with their teen, they say things such as, "She makes me crazy!" "I just want to scream!" "I could have killed him!" or "Should I survive these years . . ." It takes energy, stability, love, patience, and persistence to raise a teen.

Teens can be temperamental, rebellious, in opposition, moody, sassy, lazy, and argumentative. Indeed, some parents wonder what is wrong if their teen is being cooperative and reasonable! Yet negative behaviors are usually balanced with periods of humor, responsibility, and cooperation. Sometimes a teen behaves wonderfully outside the home, but saves their resistance for Mom or Dad. One mother said:

My children were wonderful and easy until age 13. I always wondered if there was something built in that released itself on the thirteenth birthday which was a "how to" manual on acting like a teenager. By the time they got from obnoxious into being nice again, they were eighteen and ready to fly from the nest. I never thought it was fair that after all that energy it took to get them through adolescence, I didn't get to enjoy the benefits much before they left home. However, I guess that is normal. We equip our children to leave us, and know in our hearts that it is a job well done!

Most teens are risk-takers. Most know exactly how to push your buttons, and will challenge their limits, pushing the "edge of the envelope" with all authority figures. Throughout all of this, they have an expectation that you will provide for and protect them. Your teens expect that you will be there for him or her in spite of their actions, and that you will stand by them in time of trouble. They also expect consistent rules and become confused when the rules change. In spite of their daring behaviors, they are comforted when they have firm and consistent parenting. They know the limits and consequences of their actions.

Your teen will most likely be exposed to many opportunities that are not healthy. Society lives at a fast pace. Today's teens often work a considerable number of hours, which interferes with sleep and homework. At a time of development when they actually may need more sleep, they are sleep-deprived. Meals consist of many fast foods as they eat on the go, and these are not necessarily healthy. They often stay up late, and sleep until noon when given the chance. Many teens have sexual partners at an early age, and yet they do not know much about contraception or the consequences of pregnancy. They know where to go to get cigarettes, tobacco, alcohol, marijuana, and hard drugs, and have numerous opportunities to obtain and use these. They have more money for their personal use than any other previous generation. Yet depression and suicide are more common among teens now than ever before.

You know well the challenges of parenting. You might need help to safely guide your son or daughter through adolescence. And when your child develops diabetes, there is a whole new set of concerns and expectations that arise.

Advice for Raising a Teen with Diabetes

As a parent, you have expectations of what your child will be from the time she is born. Of course, one expectation that most parents have is that their child will be healthy. When a child develops a chronic disease like diabetes, there is an adjustment that must take place as you learn to reset your perceptions of and expectations for your child. The vision of your healthy child transforms into one that includes following a diet, exercising, testing blood sugar, perhaps taking medication, and being at risk for the complications of diabetes. Suddenly you may feel that your child is vulnerable, and instinctively you may lean toward becoming overprotective. You may feel like taking on the burden of responsibility of diabetes completely.

Normally, the teen years are a time for increasing independence from parents. But when your child has diabetes, independence issues can be troublesome, as you are not sure that your child will take care of himself when apart from you. And what could be more difficult than to watch your child harm himself? You may be confused about how much compromise in diabetes care is okay in order to make your teen happy and fit in with his friends. Your child is most likely having feelings of loss and sorrow, feelings of being "different," and issues of control and trust. And, depending on the personality and temperament of your child, you may be met with cooperation or opposition as your child deals with all of these new issues. That can be tough, and it takes time and energy to deal with it. It may take some time and effort to sort out how the diagnosis of diabetes has impacted your style of parenting.

Other parents cope by going in the opposite direction; they give complete responsibility to the teen. Some parents want to hand the responsibility of self-care to their teen, yet most often the teen is not able to handle it fully. The following tips and suggestions might be helpful as you raise your teen with diabetes:

1. *Don't allow diabetes care to become a springboard for a power struggle.* It is common for the struggles and arguments of adolescence to settle upon diabetes issues. Teens have a sense of the things that are most important to you, and these become the areas of resistance. Obviously, your child's health and well-being are extremely important, and it is smart to do what you can to prevent diabetes care from being the springboard for power struggles.

If you can move your struggles to areas such as curfews, grades, homework, or dress issues, instead of diabetes issues, you may take the focus off of diabetes. One father often found himself in an argument about diabetes care issues with his daughter. They argued over blood glucose monitoring, eating candy, and taking medication. So, wisely, he instead started picking on his daughter about her eye makeup. As the fight over eye makeup escalated, the focus on diabetes issues diminished. To me he admitted, "I never did care much about her eye makeup!" As the struggles around diabetes diminished, her diabetes care improved.

2. *Be protective, but not overprotective.* As a parent, our ultimate concerns for our children are their safety, happiness, and success. However, happiness and success may very well depend on safety. You must make judgment calls based on your perceptions of what is safe or unsafe for your child. The friends they hang out with, the places they go, the hours they keep, and the use of the car are all areas where you, the parent, must decide what to allow or not allow.

Sometimes the diagnosis of diabetes makes parents anxious and confused. Where an activity may have been considered before, it now seems unsafe because of diabetes. If you are finding that you are worried about your teen, yet don't know where to draw the line in what is okay for your teen to do, it can be helpful to try to sort things out by asking yourself, "What would I be doing if he did not have diabetes?" For example, Judy was at first anxious over a decision she made not to allow her daughter (who had diabetes) to have cotton candy at the amusement park. She felt sorry for her daughter, who said her friends always could eat things she was not allowed to eat, and sometimes they teased her about it. Her daughter wanted to have fun, as it was a special day. Her daughter pestered her for the candy, even though her blood sugar was high. But then Judy realized she didn't usually allow *any* of her children to eat cotton candy (since their father was a dentist, and was concerned about their teeth), and so she closed the subject with "Our family does not eat cotton candy." After she thought about it, she felt comfortable with her decision; it had nothing to do with the diabetes, but was a household rule.

So, as you sort out issues, ask yourself, "Would I allow him/her to do that if he didn't have diabetes?" If the answer is "yes," recognize that yes, diabetes *does* complicate things, but there should be a way of safely working out anything your child with diabetes wants to do. A diabetes educator should be able to help. Of course, if the answer is "no," then it is not a diabetes issue, so leave the diabetes out of the equation.

3. *Stay involved in your child's care.* Teens want to be independent, and most parents want this as well. However, no matter how responsible your teen is in important things (such as grades, paper route, or diabetes care), there will be some areas where immaturity shows. Teens and many adults alike can have difficulty consistently maintaining their diabetes program. Most people, teens and adults alike, are not wholly adherent to their regimen. Some may do well testing and taking medication, yet struggle terribly with the meal plan. Others may do well in following dietary recommendations, yet fall off in testing their blood sugar. Your child will most likely need help from time to time. In fact, you may need to pitch in and actually do some of the tasks for your child when he is not able to do so.

In normal development, there is not steady progression from one stage to the next as teens mature. It is more of a "two steps forward, one step backward" process. Your child may do well for a while in his self-care, then slide off. You may not even notice that he has quit testing his blood unless you stay involved in his care. If he quits for any reason (priorities change, he becomes overwhelmed with something else, he is discouraged, etc.), you may need to step in and take over for a while until your child is able to resume on his own again. This does not mean that you will permanently be doing this task as your teen grows into adulthood. It is a temporary bridge to the next step. Your teen may readily take the task on again when he realizes that he has lost some independence. He also may do it more willingly when he learns there is no negotiation on the subject: It will be done no matter who has to do it!

Most people do better with tasks when they know they are going to be held accountable for their actions. In fact, our whole society is based on a system of accountability. Teens need to know that you are interested enough in their health to check the memory of their glucose meter, take them to doctor's appointments, ask what they ate, and otherwise supervise their care. They often need to be kept "on task," and that includes their diabetes care. Although you may feel like a nag, and your teen may feel as if she is being nagged, this is good parenting. You may need to say something to your teen such as, "For your whole life, I've taken care of you and done everything I could do to keep you healthy. Now that you have diabetes, I'm going to continue to do that by helping you do the things you need to do to take care of yourself. I cannot completely do it for you. But I may check the memory in your meter, or I may ask you what you ate when you were out with your friends, not to be a nag, but to care for you, who I love. Please tell me if you are having a problem sticking to your meal plan, or a problem not eating candy. Honesty is important. I want to be able to help you because I love you."

4. *Don't assume your teen is following his/her program.* Teens and adults alike may do well following their plan for a while, but then fall away from it. Sometimes you get busy and assume that your child is okay and following her routine. Parents who attend a routine doctor's visit with their teen are often surprised to learn that the numbers, dates, and times in their child's memory meter do not match what is in the daily log. It is not uncommon for numbers to be falsified or altered. Sometimes the teen is not testing, but fills in the gaps, and other times doesn't want everyone to know how high her blood sugar is. Other teens may quit taking their medication without parental knowledge. Unfortunately, good parenting involves "watchdogging."

5. *Don't forget that YOU are the parent!* Sometimes parents may be tempted to give in to the demands of their teen because it is the easier route to take. But for some things, such as health care issues, it should be made clear that there are *no negotiations and no compromises.* Your child must always take his medication, visit the doctor at three-month intervals, and monitor blood sugar.

Marcel, an African-American 14-year-old, recently sat in the doctor's office with his mother. She explained to the health care team that she had not had him checked for more than a year because he "wouldn't come." But because he hadn't been to see his doctor for a long while, his blood glucose control had deteriorated from fair to extremely poor, and he now was at significant risk for complications. The standard of care for anyone with diabetes to visit a doctor is at *three-month intervals.* By allowing her child to be in control of the situation, Marcel's mom was being negligent.

Remember that you are responsible for your child until he turns eighteen! Although your teen may be willful, you are still the parent and must stay in charge.

6. *Teach your teen that actions have consequences.* Almost any parent will tell you that sometimes your kids can wear you down. You will need to tell them what you expect from them, and the consequences if they do not meet those expectations. Then (this is the hard part) enforce the consequences. Remember the old saying, "This is going to hurt me more than it's going to hurt you!" The current term is "tough love." Sometimes our kids need to learn the hard way. For example, you may need to revoke driving privileges if Shauna quits testing her blood sugar before driving.

While teens dislike discipline and repeatedly test their limits, underneath they are grateful for limits, because without them they are lost. Teens who have few limits imposed on them easily become out of control, and that in and of itself is frightening to them. An out-of-control teen is often afraid of his own power.

Alternatively, positive reinforcement usually works better than punishment. Tell your child how pleased you are and how proud you are when she responsibly takes care of herself. Allow her to earn your trust.

7. *Be a good role model.* Our children learn all kinds of things from us, including beliefs about health care. Spirituality, understanding of our individual control over our life and destiny, and our health care practices have significant influence on those of our children. If you smoke, if you are overweight, if you drink too much alcohol, if you believe that it doesn't matter whether you take your medicine or not, if you don't exercise, if you disregard your physician's advice, you are teaching your child that it is "okay" to do so.

When it comes to dietary issues, this is especially true. Food has many meanings for us, and is connected to events and emotions. Think of all the special foods that are connected with celebrations and events, such as weddings, birthday parties, holidays, funerals, and sporting events. What do you think of when you think of food and the movies? Obviously, the answer is popcorn. Foods have strong emotional attachments. Think of the food that was special to you as you were growing up. When you see that food, even now, you probably flash back to the special time or holiday. Our eating habits are strongly connected to these emotions and also are learned behavior. You may not be able to help your teen make progress in sticking to his regimen until you are able to change your own habits and attitudes. (Sometimes our kids aren't the only ones who need an "attitude adjustment"!) Begin to try to make emotional attachments to healthy foods in your family.

If your daughter sees you down a bag of chips every time you are angry or upset, don't be surprised if she does the same. But if she sees you concerned about your health and making every attempt to eat well and maintain a healthy weight, she will be more likely to do the same. You may not make much headway with the directive "Go exercise!" But if you say, "Come and ride bikes with me," you might successfully get your teen to exercise.

8. *Take your teen for professional counseling, if necessary.* Indeed, it is difficult to adhere to a meal plan when on vacation, traveling, or partying. These events are part of life, and you and your teen will just need to do the best you can do to maintain blood sugar control during these times. However, daily dietary indiscretions can be a big problem in diabetes management. If your child struggles to eat properly at lunchtime or after school with friends, or if you are consistently finding candy wrappers in his backpack, pockets, or room, there is a problem. Most often, if the problem is addressed by you and persists, your teen may need counseling with a professional to get to the heart of the problem. Sometimes leaving the candy wrappers for you to find can be a call for help from your teen.

Sometimes talking to an objective, unbiased person in a counseling situation can be extremely helpful to struggling teens. If your child is persistently unhappy, angry, depressed, not taking care of himself, or getting into trouble at school or with police, counseling is necessary. Most often, counseling therapy can give the teen the support needed to deal with problems and move forward. Don't hesitate to talk to your teen's doctor, social worker, or health care team about a referral. Ask if they can refer you to a mental health therapist who has experience with both teens and diabetes.

9. *Listen to your teen.* While this suggestion seems so obvious, it is underused for a variety of reasons by many people. Sometimes it is difficult to catch your teen in a verbally sharing mood. You can ask a question at eight o'clock in the morning and not receive an answer, but at 7:00 P.M., when he is ready to talk, you may get a full discussion. Sometimes the best time might be at midnight! Your teen avoids intrusive questions, but underneath usually appreciates your interest.

Become adept at reading between the lines. It is not only what your teen says that is important, but also what she doesn't say. When she does talk to you, sit down and give her your full attention. Try to listen without being negative or judgmental. In order to make sure that you fully understand what she is saying to you, try to repeat it back to her. For example, after listening to your son, you may say, "Let's see. You are feeling as though your coach isn't playing you because of your diabetes, even though he hasn't said that?"

Being a good listener helps your teen know that you care, and likewise, he or she has an opportunity to vent and express feelings. It helps you, the parent, better understand your child's thoughts, feelings, and struggles. Some of the time, there will be no solutions required. The opportunity to unload may be all that is necessary.

10. *Allow your teen to work out solutions.* Sometimes the best solutions to problems that crop up may come from your teen. Encouraging your teen to solve his own problems not only can elicit creative solutions, but also gives your child a sense of control over the situation. For example, you learn that your daughter has been forgetting to take her morning metformin, because she "doesn't have time." Your message to her is that this is unacceptable, and rather than tell her what to do, instead you ask her how she is going to fix the problem. She responds by saying, "I know I have to take my pill, but I'm so tired in the morning and I don't remember it until it's too late. Maybe I can put a pill out by my toothbrush when I go to bed, so I can take it when I brush my teeth in the morning. I always brush my teeth."

11. *Find something bigger than yourself to believe in.* You will show your child how to positively deal with problems in life by investing in your spiritual side. Those who cope well with chronic illness often do so because of a strong religion or spiritual belief, and the power of prayer. This is another area where you can be a good model for your child. Even though at times our children reject our way of life for a while, what they see and learn through our own behavior can become ingrained. Our spirituality takes us outside ourselves and our own problems, and can give perspective on them. Many teens receive tremendous support from those in their church, synagogue, or youth groups.

I hope this book has given both you and your teen useful information to help manage diabetes and improve the quality of your teen's life by providing practical tips and insights into the problems that you encounter. Living with diabetes, at least for now, is a lifelong process, and you will not be perfect at it all of the time. Remember to look at the big picture, not the daily frustrations. Hopefully, someday we will have a cure, but until then, do the best you can do. If your teen is interested in learning, even as much as reading this book, that is a great first step!

10

Parting Thoughts

I am very proud of the teens in Chapter 8 who took the time and energy to have a discussion about diabetes. It was obvious to me after talking with them how difficult it is to grow up and have diabetes, whether it is type 1 or type 2. Also surprising to me is the general comment from those with type 2 that they are grateful they don't have type 1! They see having to take insulin as something to be dreaded. (On the other hand, teens with type 1 often are grateful that they can take insulin to cover extra food or a sweet dessert and, unless they are overweight, can eat in a less restricted way.)

The issues of most concern for teens with type 2 diabetes are about weight, food restrictions, and people, especially parents, who act like the "food police." This is a concern that parents and health care professionals alike should heed. You can be supportive in the effort without nagging. This is hard to do sometimes, so if you are a teen reading this, you may want to think about how you can guide your loving naggers into more productive and positive behaviors. They are trying to be helpful and are concerned about your well-being. Often a parent does not know how to help, so you must teach them what is helpful to you and what isn't.

Over time, most teens feel as though they have a handle on what they need to do for their diabetes care. Most of them have accepted their diabetes as a way of life even though they don't like it. As another patient told me, "My grandma says, 'We all have our cross to bear.' "

It was also gratifying to learn that many of the teens who deal with type 2 diabetes, and deal with it well, have a strong faith and religious affiliations. Their spiritual lives have helped them deal with misfortune in a very positive way. If you don't have a spiritual life, you may want to think about how you could connect with someone who will introduce you to religion and prayer. If you do have a spiritual life, use it to deal with more difficult things in your life.

Last, I was impressed that teens with type 2 have an understanding about the effects of diabetes on their future. Yes, they are concerned about their health, and there is a sense that they are afraid because, as Bridget put it, "I feel like I'm doing something wrong." They have a rough time sticking to their diabetes program and feel vulnerable when they fall off. They feel guilty when they go off their meal plan and worry that they may be hurting themselves. Even though they understand that diabetes is for life, and so there is no expectation they will do everything perfectly, there seems to be a feeling that when they slip off their program, they have done wrong.

They know that complications can occur, and yet seem to look forward to better ways of treating diabetes in the future. In fact, research has come a long way, and so has the technology of treating diabetes. In the many years since I personally was diagnosed with diabetes, the progress has been astounding. To give you an example, in 1982 I got my first blood glucose meter. It weighed about 5 pounds, had to be plugged into the wall, was bigger than a phone, required a squirt water bottle, timer, and blotting paper, and took over two minutes! The finger lancets were huge and made big cuts in the fingers, and you needed a big drop of blood. Even more of a concern is that the results were not always accurate. Less than twenty years later we have credit-card size, five-second meters that require a tiny amount of blood and are quite accurate. Next will be noninvasive meters!

So be optimistic about the future of diabetes research and

technology. No, we don't have a cure yet, but there are billions of dollars being spent today toward that end. It will come, and hopefully in our lifetime. At the least, there will be better ways of treating diabetes in the future. So hang in there and stick to your program. Try to be patient and stay well so that when the cure *does* come, you won't already have done irreparable damage!

Glossary

adrenaline (epinephrine) is a hormone that your body makes when you are stressed or frightened. It can cause blood sugar to go up.

autoimmune disease is caused when fighting cells, or antibodies, attack healthy body tissues. In Type 1 diabetes, the cells that make insulin are destroyed.

beta cells are the cells that make insulin.

blood glucose is a measurement of how much sugar is in your blood. It is measured in milligrams per deciliter (mg/dl). A normal blood glucose is 70–120 mg/dl.

blood glucose meter is a device for measuring how much sugar is in the blood.

calorie is a measure of the energy it takes to use food. Calories come from carbohydrate, protein, and fat. Calories that are not used as energy are stored as fat.

capillary is a very tiny blood vessel. When you stick your finger to see what your blood glucose is, you measure capillary blood.

carbohydrates are starches found in grains, fruits, vegetables, and milk products. Protein has a little carbohydrate. Carbohydrate must be turned into glucose in order to be used by the body.

cells are the smallest unit of life.

chronic disease is one that is long-lasting. Diabetes is a chronic illness because it does not yet have a cure.

dehydration is a state of not enough fluids in the body. High blood sugar can cause dehydration.

diabetes is a disease where insulin is either not made or not used properly.

dialysis is a way that machines remove wastes from the blood when the kidneys don't work properly. Kidney disease is a complication that can occur after many years of diabetes, and is most common in people with poorly controlled blood glucose levels.

dietitian is a licensed health care worker who helps people to stay well through healthy eating.

digestion is the process where the food you eat is turned into substances that the body can use.

endocrinologist is a medical doctor who specializes in the treatment of diseases of the glands that make hormones.

epinephrine see adrenaline

fats are a source of energy for the body. Fats can be saturated (found mostly in animal products) and unsaturated (found mostly in plants). High levels of fat in the blood can cause heart disease and stroke.

fiber is the part of foods that adds bulk that cannot be digested. Foods and vegetables are high in fiber.

fructose is a form of sugar found in fruit.

glucagon is a hormone produced by the pancreas that raises blood glucose. An injection of glucagon is the treatment for severe symptoms of low blood glucose.

glucose is a form of sugar. Food is turned into glucose during digestion. It is what body cells need for energy.

glycated hemoglobin (HbAlc) is an indication of what the average blood glucose level has been over the past two months.

hormones are chemical substances released by a gland into the bloodstream. Insulin is a hormone.

hyperglycemia is a high level of glucose in the blood. Signs include increased thirst, frequent urination, tiredness, and blurred vision.

hypoglycemia is a low level of glucose in the blood. Signs include sweating, shakiness, hunger, dizziness, irritability, and confusion.

insulin is a hormone produced by the beta cells of the pancreas. It helps the body to use glucose for energy.

insulin resistance is found in type 2 diabetes when the body does not efficiently use the insulin being made. This can be caused by obesity and sedentary behaviors, and is made worse by the hormones produced during the teen years.

islets of Langerhans are clusters of cells in the pancreas that produce insulin.

juvenile-onset diabetes, or insulin-dependent diabetes is a former name for what is now called type 1 diabetes.

ketone is a waste product made by the body when it burns fat for energy.

ketoacidosis is a condition that occurs when ketones build up in the blood, causing it to become acidic. Signs are labored breathing, fruity-smelling breath, dehydration, and ketones in the urine and blood. Ketoacidosis should be promptly treated. It usually occurs in people with type 1 diabetes.

kidney is one of two organs that filter waste products from the blood. Poor diabetes control and high blood pressure can damage kidneys.

logbooks are one way of keeping records of blood glucose levels, ketones, exercise, and food.

maturity-onset diabetes, or non-insulin-dependent diabetes is now called type 2 diabetes.

metabolism refers to the changes caused by hormones, chemicals, and physical functioning, which allow cells to live and grow.

nephropathy is a kidney disease that can be a complication of diabetes.

neuropathy is a nerve disease that can be a complication of diabetes.

ophthalmologist is a medical doctor (M.D.) who specializes in the care of eye disease.

optometrist is a specialist who is licensed to examine eyes and prescribe lenses.

pancreas is the organ that produces insulin, digestive juices, and other hormones.

protein is a building block of metabolism and a source of energy.

psychiatrist is a medical doctor (M.D.) who specializes in treating mental illness and can prescribe medications for it.

psychologist is a health care professional trained in counseling and the treatment of problems that cause mental and emotional illness.

retinopathy is an eye complication of diabetes.

sucrose is table sugar.

type 1 diabetes is an autoimmune disease where the pancreas does not make insulin at all.

type 2 diabetes is a disease where the body may not make enough insulin and cannot properly use the insulin available.

Index

Other Works by Jean Betschart-Roemer

For more information visit the author's website, *www.diabetes. fyi.net*

American Diabetes Association Guide to Raising a Child with Diabetes, 2nd ed., with Linda Siminerio, American Diabetes Association, 2000.

Diabetes Care for Babies, Toddlers and Preschoolers, John Wiley and Sons, 1999.

In Control: A Guide for Teens with Diabetes, with Susan Thom, John Wiley and Sons, 1995.

It's Time to Learn About Diabetes Workbook, John Wiley and Sons, 1995.

It's Time to Learn About Diabetes Video, available from the author, 1992.

It's Time to Learn about Diabetes CD-Rom, available from the author, 2001.

A Magic Ride in Foozbah-Land, John Wiley and Sons (audiotape available from the author), 1995.

50 Ways to Manage Your Diabetes, Publications International, 2000.

About the Author

Jean Betschart-Roemer is a Certified Registered Pediatric Nurse Practitioner and Certified Diabetes Educator in the Department of Diabetes, Endocrinology, and Metabolism of Children's Hospital of Pittsburgh. She has a master's degree in parent–child nursing and a Master of Science in Nursing in pediatric health promotion and development from the University of Pittsburgh.

She is a past president of the American Association of Diabetes Educators and a past recipient of the American Diabetes Association's Outstanding Health Professional Educator Award. She is active as a diabetes camp volunteer and currently edits the "For Parents" series of the magazine *Diabetes Self-Management.*